T0226828

Waldenström Macroglobulinemia

Editors

JORGE J. CASTILLO
EFSTATHIOS KASTRITIS
STEVEN P. TREON

HEMATOLOGY/ONCOLOGY
CLINICS OF NORTH AMERICA

www.hemonc.theclinics.com

Consulting Editors
GEORGE P. CANELLOS
H. FRANKLIN BUNN

October 2018 • Volume 32 • Number 5

ELSEVIER

1600 John F. Kennedy Boulevard • Suite 1800 • Philadelphia, Pennsylvania, 19103-2899

http://www.theclinics.com

HEMATOLOGY/ONCOLOGY CLINICS OF NORTH AMERICA Volume 32, Number 5
October 2018 ISSN 0889-8588, ISBN 13: 978-0-323-64127-2

Editor: Stacy Eastman
Developmental Editor: Kristen Helm

Hematology/Oncology Clinics (ISSN 0889-8588) is published bimonthly by Elsevier Inc., 360 Park Avenue South, New York, NY 10010-1710. Months of issue are February, April, June, August, October, and December. Business and Editorial Offices: 1600 John F. Kennedy Blvd., Ste. 1800, Philadelphia, PA 19103–2899. Customer Service Office: 3251 Riverport Lane, Maryland Heights, MO 63043. Periodicals postage paid at New York, NY and at additional mailing offices. Subscription prices are $413.00 per year (domestic individuals), $787.00 per year (domestic institutions), $100.00 per year (domestic students/residents), $471.00 per year (Canadian individuals), $974.00 per year (Canadian institutions) $536.00 per year (international individuals), $974.00 per year (international institutions), and $255.00 per year (international and Canadian students/residents). International air speed delivery is included in all Clinics subscription prices. All prices are subject to change without notice. **POSTMASTER:** Send address changes to Hematology/Oncology Clinics of North America, Elsevier Health Sciences Division, Subscription Customer Service, 3251 Riverport Lane, Maryland Heights, MO 63043. Customer Service (orders, claims, online, change of address): Elsevier Health Sciences Division, Subscription **Customer Service, 3251 Riverport Lane, Maryland Heights, MO 63043. Tel: 1-800-654-2452 (U.S. and Canada); 314-447-8871 (outside U.S. and Canada). Fax: 314-447-8029. E-mail: journalscustomerservice-usa@elsevier.com (for print support); journalsonlinesupport-usa@elsevier.com (for online support).**

Reprints. For copies of 100 or more, of articles in this publication, please contact the Commercial Reprints Department, Elsevier Inc., 360 Park Avenue South, New York, New York 10010-1710; Tel.: 212-633-3874, Fax: 212-633-3820, E-mail: reprints@elsevier.com.

Hematology/Oncology Clinics of North America is covered in MEDLINE/PubMed (Index Medicus), EMBASE/ Excerpta Medica, and BIOSIS.

Contributors

CONSULTING EDITORS

GEORGE P. CANELLOS, MD
William Rosenberg Professor of Medicine, Department of Medical Oncology, Dana-Farber Cancer Institute, Boston, Massachusetts, USA

H. FRANKLIN BUNN, MD
Professor of Medicine, Division of Hematology, Brigham and Women's Hospital, Harvard Medical School, Boston, Massachusetts, USA

EDITORS

JORGE J. CASTILLO, MD
Clinical Director, Bing Center for Waldenström's Macroglobulinemia, Dana-Farber Cancer Institute, Assistant Professor, Department of Medicine, Harvard Medical School, Boston, Massachusetts, USA

EFSTATHIOS KASTRITIS, MD
Associate Professor, Department of Clinical Therapeutics, National and Kapodistrian University of Athens School of Medicine, Athens, Greece; Bing Center for Waldenström's Macroglobulinemia, Athens, Attica, Greece

STEVEN P. TREON, MD, PhD
Director, Bing Center for Waldenström's Macroglobulinemia, Dana-Farber Cancer Institute, Professor, Department of Medicine, Harvard Medical School, Boston, Massachusetts, USA

AUTHORS

RANJANA H. ADVANI, MD
Saul A. Rosenberg Professor of Lymphoma, Division of Oncology, Department of Medicine, Stanford University, Stanford Cancer Institute, Stanford, California, USA

STEPHEN M. ANSELL, MD, PhD
Division of Hematology, Mayo Clinic, Rochester, Minnesota, USA

KIMON V. ARGYROPOULOS, MD
Immunology Program, Memorial Sloan Kettering Cancer Center, New York, New York, USA

CHRISTIAN BUSKE, MD
Comprehensive Cancer Center Ulm, Institute of Experimental Cancer Research, University Hospital Ulm, Ulm, Germany

JORGE J. CASTILLO, MD
Clinical Director, Bing Center for Waldenström's Macroglobulinemia, Dana-Farber Cancer Institute, Assistant Professor, Department of Medicine, Harvard Medical School, Boston, Massachusetts, USA

MELETIOS A. DIMOPOULOS, MD
Department of Clinical Therapeutics, National and Kapodistrian University of Athens School of Medicine, Athens, Greece

ANDRES DOMINGUEZ, MD
Department of Internal Medicine, Fundación Valle del Lili, CES University, Cali, Colombia

AMAIA GASCUE, BS
Department of Immunology, Clínica Universidad de Navarra, Pamplona, Spain

ZACHARY R. HUNTER, PhD
Bing Center for Waldenström's Macroglobulinemia, Dana-Farber Cancer Institute, Department of Medicine, Harvard Medical School, Boston, Massachusetts, USA

SHAHRZAD JALALI, PhD
Division of Hematology, Mayo Clinic, Rochester, Minnesota, USA

EFSTATHIOS KASTRITIS, MD
Associate Professor, Department of Clinical Therapeutics, National and Kapodistrian University of Athens School of Medicine, Athens, Greece; Bing Center for Waldenström's Macroglobulinemia, Athens, Attica, Greece

CHARALAMPIA KYRIAKOU, MD, PhD
Consultant Haematologist, Department of Haematology, University College London, London, United Kingdom

XAVIER LELEU, MD, PhD
Department of Hematology, Hospital of the Miletrie, CHU of Poitiers, Poitiers, France

M. LIA, MD
Department of Medicine, Lymphoma Service, Memorial Sloan Kettering Cancer Center, New York, New York, USA

XIA LIU, MD
Bing Center for Waldenström's Macroglobulinemia, Dana-Farber Cancer Institute, Boston, Massachusetts, USA

MARION MAGIEROWICZ, Pharm D
Laboratory of Hematology, Biology and Pathology Center, CHU of Lille, Lille, France

MARY L. McMASTER, MD
Clinical Genetics Branch, Division of Cancer Epidemiology and Genetics, National Cancer Institute, National Institutes of Health, US Department of Health and Human Services, Bethesda, Maryland, USA; Commissioned Corps of the US Public Health Service, US Department of Health and Human Services, Washington, DC, USA

JUANA MERINO, MD, PhD
Department of Immunology, Clínica Universidad de Navarra, Pamplona, Spain

BRUNO PAIVA, PhD
Clinica Universidad de Navarra, Centre for Applied Medical Research (CIMA), Instituto de Investigación Sanitaria de Navarra (IDISNA), Pamplona, Spain; CIBERONC, Spain

STÉPHANIE POULAIN, Pharm D, PhD
Laboratory of Hematology, Biology and Pathology Center, CHU of Lille, Lille, France

MICHAEL A. SPINNER, MD
Hematology/Oncology Fellow, Division of Oncology, Department of Medicine, Stanford University, Stanford Cancer Institute, Stanford, California, USA

CÉCILE TOMOWIAK, MD
Department of Hematology, Hospital of the Miletrie, CHU of Poitiers, Poitiers, France

STEVEN P. TREON, MD, PhD
Director, Bing Center for Waldenström's Macroglobulinemia, Dana-Farber Cancer Institute, Professor, Department of Medicine, Harvard Medical School, Boston, Massachusetts, USA

GAURAV VARMA, MD, MSPH
Department of Medicine, NewYork-Presbyterian Hospital/Weill Cornell Medicine, New York, New York, USA

LIAN XU, MA
Bing Center for Waldenström's Macroglobulinemia, Dana-Farber Cancer Institute, Boston, Massachusetts, USA

GUANG YANG, PhD
Bing Center for Waldenström's Macroglobulinemia, Dana-Farber Cancer Institute, Department of Medicine, Harvard Medical School, Boston, Massachusetts, USA

Contents

Next-generation sequencing has revealed recurring somatic mutations in Waldenström macroglobulinemia (WM). Common mutations include MYD88 (95%–97%), as well as CXCR4 (30%–40%), ARID1A (17%), and CD79B (8%–15%), which are typically found in patients with MYD88 mutation. The genomic findings provide important insights into the pathogenesis, prognostication, and treatment outcome in WM. The authors discuss the genomic landscape of WM and the impact of underlying genomics on disease presentation, transcriptional changes, treatment outcome, and overall survival.

Waldenström macroglobulinemia is a rare indolent B-cell lymphoma. Whole-exome sequencing studies have improved our knowledge of the Waldenström macroglobulinemia mutational landscape. The MYD88 L265P mutation is present in nearly 90% of patients with Waldenström macroglobulinemia. *CXCR4* mutations are identified in approximately 30% of MYD88L265P cases and have been associated with ibrutinib resistance in clinical trials. Mutations in *CD79B, ARID1a*, or *TP53* were described at lower frequency. Deciphering the earliest initiating lesions and identifying the molecular alterations leading to disease progression currently represent important goals in the future to identify the most relevant targets for precision therapy in Waldenström macroglobulinemia.

Multiparameter flow cytometry (MFC) is valuable in the diagnosis and monitoring of most hematologic malignancies. Although the assessment of cellular infiltrates in Waldenström macroglobulinemia (WM) relies on morphology and immunohistochemistry grounds, there is evidence pointing to the clinical significance of MFC in this disease. Herein, the authors review immunophenotypic patterns of B-cell development, the antigen profile of the WM clone and its normal B-cell counterpart, the clinical applicability of MFC in the differential diagnosis of immunoglobulin M–secreting lymphoproliferative disorders and monoclonal gammopathies, and its

used. Rituximab, cyclophosphamide, doxorubicin, vincristine, and prednisone (R-CHOP) is a highly effective but potentially neurotoxic regimen. Dexamethasone, rituximab, and cyclophosphamide (DRC) induces long responses and has a favorable toxicity profile. Bendamustine was shown to be among the most potent chemotherapeutics in combination with rituximab. Future studies must define the role of alkylating agents, which compete with highly effective chemotherapy-free targeted therapies.

Waldenström macroglobulinemia (WM) is an indolent low-grade non-Hodgkin lymphoma characterized by bone marrow infiltration by lympho-plasmacytic cells and associated clonal IgM paraproteinemia. Recent insights into the biology and genomic characteristics of WM have provided a further platform for more targeted therapies. Despite the high response rates and better depth and duration of responses, the disease remains incurable. This article focuses on use of the high-dose therapy with either autologous or allogeneic hematopoietic stem cell transplant.

Recent advances in the understanding of Waldenström macroglobuli-nemia (WM) biology have paved the way for the development of a plethora of novel therapeutic strategies. The success of ibrutinib in WM has shifted treatment paradigms away from conventional chemoimmunotherapy ap-proaches. Recognition of high-risk genomic subgroups, as well as mech-anisms of acquired resistance to ibrutinib, has led to targeting of additional pathways. In this article, the authors review ongoing and emerging trials of novel therapies in WM that target the B-cell receptor pathway beyond ibru-tinib, toll-like receptor pathway, chemokine signaling, apoptotic pathway, chromatin remodeling, protein transport, the immune microenvironment, and CD19-directed immunotherapy.

HEMATOLOGY/ONCOLOGY
CLINICS OF NORTH AMERICA

ISSUE OF RELATED INTEREST

Surgical Pathology Clinics, March 2016 (Vol. 9, Issue 1)
Hematopathology
Yuri Fedoriw, *Editor*
Available at: http://www.surgpath.theclinics.com/

THE CLINICS ARE AVAILABLE ONLINE!
Access your subscription at:
www.theclinics.com

Preface

Waldenström Macroglobulinemia: Lessons Learned from Basic and Clinical Research

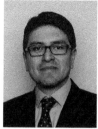 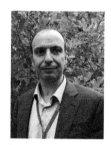 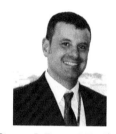

Jorge J. Castillo, MD   Efstathios Kastritis, MD   Steven P. Treon, MD, PhD

Editors

Waldenström macroglobulinemia (WM) was first described by Dr Jan G. Waldenström over 70 years ago. WM was initially reported as a syndrome characterized by anemia and symptoms of hyperviscosity due to a large protein or "macroglobulin" in patients with an incipient myelomatosis in the bone marrow. Over the last 7 decades, our understanding on the genomics, biology, diagnostic criteria, and treatment approaches has deepened thanks to the tireless efforts of men and women dedicated to investigating WM. As such, WM is now recognized as an immunoglobulin M–secreting lymphoplasmacytic lymphoma that involves the bone marrow, and other organs, and is characterized by recurrent somatic mutations in MYD88 and CXCR4 in 90% and 40% of patients, respectively. For this issue of the *Hematology/Oncology Clinics of North America*, the editors have put together an all-star team of basic and clinical researchers to provide the readers with an issue focused on the most recent developments in WM. Among other topics, of great interest are in-depth discussions of the genomic basis of WM. Specifically, Dr Steven Treon and Dr Stéphanie Poulain review not only the identification of the MYD88 L265P and CXCR4 mutations, respectively, but also the translational importance and clinical applicability of these mutations. Dr Bruno Paiva delves into the current understanding of the role of flow cytometry on the progression of WM and as a potential tool for identifying the true WM stem cell. Dr Stephen Ansell discusses the role of the microenvironment on the development and sustainment of WM. Dr Mary McMaster provides additional insights into familial WM. Dr Jorge Castillo discusses the appropriate initial evaluation of patients with WM. With regards to treatment options, Dr Christian Buske focuses on the experience accumulated with alkylating agents, and Dr Efstathios Kastritis reviews the available data on proteasome inhibitors. Dr Jorge Castillo discusses the role of monoclonal antibodies; Dr M. Lia

Hematol Oncol Clin N Am 32 (2018) xiii–xiv
https://doi.org/10.1016/j.hoc.2018.07.001
0889-8588/18/© 2018 Published by Elsevier Inc.

hemonc.theclinics.com

Palomba provides an update on the use of Bruton tyrosine kinase inhibitors, and Dr Charalampia Kyriakou looks into the current experience with hematopoietic stem cell transplantation in patients with WM. Finally, Dr Ranjana Advani takes us into uncharted waters with a review on novel treatment approaches for patients with WM. We hope the current issue of *Hematology/Oncology Clinics of North America* focusing on WM will serve as a point of reference for researchers and clinicians alike.

Jorge J. Castillo, MD
Bing Center for Waldenström's Macroglobulinemia
Dana-Farber Cancer Institute
Harvard Medical School
450 Brookline Avenue, M221
Boston, MA 02215, USA

Efstathios Kastritis, MD
Department of Clinical Therapeutics
National and Kapodistrian University of Athens
80 Vasilissis Sofias Avenue
Athens, Attica 11528, Greece

Steven P. Treon, MD, PhD
Bing Center for Waldenström's Macroglobulinemia
Dana-Farber Cancer Institute
Harvard Medical School
450 Brookline Avenue, M548
Boston, MA 02215, USA

E-mail addresses:
JorgeJ_Castillo@dfci.harvard.edu (J.J. Castillo)
ekastritis@med.uoa.gr (E. Kastritis)
steven_treon@dfci.harvard.edu (S.P. Treon)

Genomic Landscape of Waldenström Macroglobulinemia

Steven P. Treon, MD, PhD[a,b,*], Lian Xu, MA[a], Xia Liu, MD[a],
Zachary R. Hunter, PhD[a,b], Guang Yang, PhD[a,b],
Jorge J. Castillo, MD[a,b]

KEYWORDS

- Genomics • Waldenström macroglobulinemia • MYD88 • CXCR4 • Pathogenesis
- Treatment

KEY POINTS

- Next-generation sequencing has revealed recurring somatic mutations in Waldenström macroglobulinemia (WM).
- Common mutations include MYD88 (95%–97%), CXCR4 (30%–40%), ARID1A (17%), and CD79B (8%–15%), which are typically found in MYD88-mutated patients.
- The genomic findings provide important insights into the pathogenesis, prognostication, and treatment outcome in WM.

INTRODUCTION

Next-generation sequencing has identified recurring somatic mutations in myeloid differentiation primary response 88 (MYD88), as well as C-X-C chemokine receptor type 4 (CXCR4), AT-rich interactive domain 1A (ARID1A), and cluster of differentiation (CD)79, along with copy number alterations impacting regulatory genes that affect nuclear factor kappa-B (NFKB), Bruton tyrosine kinase (BTK), B-cell lymphoma 2 (BCL2), and apoptosis in chromosome 6q, and elsewhere.[1] Although most patients with Waldenström macroglobulinemia (WM) (95%) carry an MYD88 mutation, those that do not show a more aggressive disease course and many somatic mutations that overlap with those found in diffuse large B-cell lymphoma (DLBCL).[2,3] Herein we discuss the genomic landscape of WM, and the impact of underlying genomics on disease presentation, transcriptional changes, treatment outcome, and overall survival.

[a] Bing Center for Waldenström's Macroglobulinemia, Dana-Farber Cancer Institute, Boston, MA 02215, USA; [b] Department of Medicine, Harvard Medical School, Boston, MA 02215, USA
* Corresponding author. Bing Center for Waldenström's Macroglobulinemia, Dana-Farber Cancer Institute, M547, 450 Brookline Avenue, Boston, MA 02215.
E-mail address: steven_treon@dfci.harvard.edu

Hematol Oncol Clin N Am 32 (2018) 745–752
https://doi.org/10.1016/j.hoc.2018.05.003
0889-8588/18/© 2018 Elsevier Inc. All rights reserved.

MUTATIONS IN MYD88

A recurring somatic mutation in MYD88 (MYD88 L265P) was identified in 91% of patients with WM by paired tumor/normal whole-genome sequencing, and subsequently confirmed by Sanger sequencing and allele-specific polymerase chain reaction (PCR) assays.[4–9] By sensitive allele-specific PCR testing, MYD88 L265P was expressed in 93% to 97% of patients with WM, including sorted CD19+ CD138− B cells, as well as CD19− CD138+ plasma cells that make up the malignant clone in WM. In addition, non-L265P MYD88 mutations have also been identified in patients with WM, including S219C, M232T, and S243N, although their expression estimates are much lower at 1% to 2%.[8] MYD88 mutations also are detectable in 50% to 80% of immunoglobulin (Ig)M but not IgG or IgA monoclonal gammopathy of undetermined significance (MGUS), suggesting an early oncogenic role for WM pathogenesis.[5–7] Patients with IgM MGUS with mutated MYD88, as well as a higher mutated allele burden for those who are MYD88 mutated, may identify those patients with IgM MGUS at higher risk of progression to WM.[5,10]

The MYD88 L265P mutation also can be detected by allele-specific PCR in peripheral blood samples, particularly in treatment-naïve patients with WM. Prior therapy with B-cell–depleting agents though can greatly decrease the detection of MYD88 L265P in peripheral blood samples.[11] In addition, MYD88 L265P can be found in cerebrospinal fluid and pleural effusions, providing a means of detecting WM disease in patients with central nervous system or pleural disease involvement.[12,13]

Structural events on chromosome 3p can increase the allele burden of mutated MYD88 in 12% to 13% of untreated patients, and upward to 25% of previously treated patients, and segue with CXCR4 mutations in the latter population.[4,8] Deletions of the wild-type (WT) MYD88 allele, and amplifications of the mutant MYD88 allele, have been observed, although acquired uniparental disomy events are the most common reason for homozygous mutated MYD88.[4,8,14] The clinical significance of these structural changes remains to be clarified, but may be relevant to time from diagnosis and ibrutinib response.

The presence or absence of MYD88 mutations discerns 2 distinct populations of patients with WM. Patients lacking MYD88 mutations show histologically similar disease to MYD88-mutated patients but present with more aggressive disease, manifested in decreased overall survival, higher risk of disease transformation, and lack of response to ibrutinib (discussed later in this article).[2,15]

MYD88 is an adaptor protein that interacts with the Toll-like receptor (TLR) and interleukin (IL)-1 receptor families, and undergoes dimerization on receptor activation. The dimerization of MYD88 provides a scaffold for the recruitment of other proteins to a "Myddosome" that triggers downstream signaling leading to NFKB activation (**Fig. 1**).[16] Both IL-1 receptor-associated kinase 1 (IRAK1)/IRAK4 and BTK are components of the "Myddosome" and trigger NFKB independent of IRAK1/IRAK4.[17,18] Recruitment and activation of the IRAK and BTK molecules can be blocked by either knockdown or inhibition of MYD88 that leads to apoptosis of MYD88-mutated WM cells.[17–19] Mutated MYD88 can also upregulate transcription of HCK, an SRC family member that is normally downregulated in late stages of B-cell ontogeny.[20] Mutated MYD88 can also transactivate HCK through production of IL-6. Activated HCK in turn triggers prosurvival signaling of mutated WM cells through BTK, PI3K/AKT, and mitogen-activated protein kinase (MAPK)/extracellular signal-regulated kinase (ERK)1/2.[20] Both BTK and HCK are potent targets of ibrutinib, which has shown remarkable activity in patients with MYD88-mutated WM.[15,20]

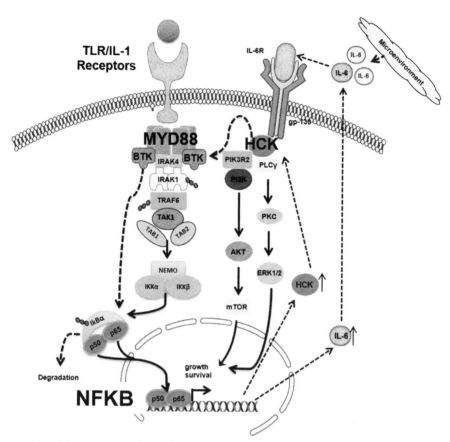

Fig. 1. Mutated MYD88-related signaling in WM. Mutated MYD88 transactivates NFKB through divergent pathways that include IRAK1/IRAK4 and BTK. Mutated MYD88 also triggers transcription and activation of the SRC family member HCK. Activated HCK can then trigger BTK, AKT, and ERK1/2-mediated progrowth and survival signaling in WM cells.

MUTATIONS IN C-X-C CHEMOKINE RECEPTOR TYPE 4

Mutations in the C-terminal domain of CXCR4 are present in up to 40% of patients with WM, and although they almost always occur with MYD88 mutations, some patients with WT MYD88 can also express these mutations.[2,21–24] CXCR4 mutations are essentially unique to WM, as they have not been described so far in other diseases, with the exception of a few marginal zone B-cell lymphoma (MZL) and activated B-cell-like (ABC) DLBCL cases. Germline mutations in the C-terminal domain of CXCR4 are also present in patients with WHIM (autosomal dominant warts, hypogammaglobulinemia, infection, and myelokathexis) syndrome.[25] In patients with WHIM syndrome, activation of CXCR4 by its ligand CXCL12 causes extended chemotactic signaling and neutrophil sequestration in the bone marrow (myelokathexis) and impairment of lymphocyte development.[25] In WM, more than 30 different nonsense and frameshift mutations in the C-terminal domain of CXCR4 have been described. Mutations in the C-terminal domain of CXCR4 lead to loss of regulatory serines, which undergo phosphorylation following CXCR4 receptor activation by CXCL12.[25] With the rest of this g-protein–coupled receptor (GPCR) left intact, mutated CXCR4 remains fully competent in downstream signaling via g-proteins and beta-arrestins, resulting in the constitutive PI3K/AKT and MAPK/ERK1/2 signaling. Despite the autonomous prosurvival signaling of CXCR4 mutations, inhibition of MYD88 led to apoptosis of both WT and mutated CXCR4-expressing WM cells, suggesting primacy of mutated MYD88 survival signaling in WM.[26]

Unlike MYD88, CXCR4 mutant clonality is highly variable. Multiple CXCR4 mutations also can exist within individual patients, which occur in separate clones or are present as compound heterozygous events.[22] The subclonal nature of CXCR4 mutations relative to MYD88 suggests that these mutations occur after MYD88, although this is likely to be an early event in WM pathogenesis given their detection in patients with IgM MGUS.[22,23] Clonal 6q deletions, which are found in 40% to 50% of patients with WM, appear exclusive of CXCR4.[27]

Like MYD88, the presence of CXCR4 somatic mutations can impact disease presentation in WM. Patients with CXCR4 mutations present with a significantly lower rate of adenopathy, and those with CXCR4 nonsense mutations have increased bone marrow disease, serum IgM levels, and/or symptomatic hyperviscosity. Despite differences in clinical presentation, CXCR4 mutations do not appear to adversely impact overall survival in WM.[2,28]

In vitro modeling of WM cells transduced with mutated CXCR4 showed increased drug resistance in the presence of CXCL12 to multiple therapeutics, including bendamustine, fludarabine, bortezomib, idelalisib, and ibrutinib.[26,29,30] Importantly, these studies showed that resistance mediated by mutated CXCR4 could be reversed by use of CXCR4 blocking agents, and a clinical trial examining the CXCR4 antagonist ulocuplumab along with ibrutinib has been initiated in CXCR4-mutated WM.

OTHER RECURRING MUTATIONS

Somatic mutations in ARID1A are present in 17% of patients with WM, nonsense, and frameshift variants.[1] Patients with ARID1A and MYD88 L265P mutations showed greater bone marrow disease involvement, and lower hemoglobin and platelet count. ARID1A and its frequently deleted homologue ARID1B (discussed later in this article) are on chromosome 6q.[1,27] Both are switch/sucrose nonfermentable (SWI/SNF) family members, and serve as chromatin-remodeling genes, thereby modulating gene regulation. Although still poorly understood, ARID1A can modulate TP53, and is thought to act as an epigenetic tumor suppressor in ovarian cancer.[31–33] CD79A and CD79B can be found in 8% to 12% of patients with WM. Both are components of the B-cell receptor (BCR) pathway, and can form heterodimers with each other.[33,34] The CD79A/B heterodimer associates with the immunoglobulin heavy chain required for cell surface expression of BCR, and BCR induced signaling.[33,34] Activating mutations in the immunotyrosine-based activation motif (ITAM) of CD79A and CD79B have been reported in ABC DLBCL, and trigger spleen tyrosine kinase (SYK), phospholipase Cγ2 (PLCγ2), and BTK. The role of BCR in WM pathogenesis remains to be clarified, although enhanced BCR signaling was observed in WM cells stimulated with BCR activating agents.[35] Deletions of LYN that are found in 70% of patients with WM could contribute to hyperresponsive BCR signaling as informed by lyn−/− transgenic mice.[36] Although mutations in both CD79A and CD79B are mainly found in patients with MYD88 mutation, a CD79B mutation was observed in a patient with MYD88 WT WM.[3,23,37] In one study, CD79A and CD79B were nearly exclusive to CXCR4 mutations, suggesting that 2 distinct MYD88 mutated populations may exist with WM.[23] In a small series of patients with WM, the coexpression of CD79B and MYD88 mutations associated with disease transformation.[38]

MUTATIONS IN MYD88 WILD-TYPE WALDENSTRÖM MACROGLOBULINEMIA

A small number of patients with WM (5%) lack mutations in MYD88, including non-L265P mutations. Their disease course is marked by an increased risk of disease transformation and shorter overall survival.[2] Moreover, these patients show little activity to the BTK inhibitor ibrutinib. These findings point to fundamental differences in underlying genomics. Whole-exome sequencing identified somatic mutations in patients with MYD88 WT WM that are predicted to trigger NFKB (TBL1XR1, PTPN13, MALT1, BCL10, NFKB1, NFKB2, NFKBIB, NFKBIZ, and UDRL1F), impart epigenomic dysregulation (KMT2D, KMT2C, KDM6A), or impair DNA damage repair (TP53, ATM, and TRRAP).[3] Predicted NFKB activating mutations were downstream of BTK, and many overlapped with somatic mutations found in DLBCL.[39,40]

Transcriptome studies revealed a distinctive transcriptional profile in patients with MYD88 WT WM, although most differentially expressed genes overlapped with those found in MYD88-mutated WM.[3] These findings are likely to explain many of the uniform characteristics shared among patients with WM, regardless of their underlying MYD88 mutation status.

COPY NUMBER ALTERATIONS

Copy number alterations are common in patients with MYD88-mutated WM, and involve both chromosome 6q, and non–chromosome 6q regions.[27,41] In chromosome 6q, loss of genes that modulate NFKB activity (TNFAIP3, HIVEP2), BCL2 (BCLAF1), apoptosis (FOXO3), BTK (IBTK), plasma cell differentiation (PRDM1), and ARID1B occur. Non–chromosome 6q genes that are commonly deleted include ETV6, a transcription repressor; BTG1, that often is deleted in DLBCL, and associated with glucocorticoid resistance in acute lymphocytic leukemia; as well as LYN, a kinase that regulates BCR signaling. PRDM2 and TOP1 that participate in TP53-related signaling are also deleted in many patients with WM.[41] In contrast to $MYD88^{MUT}$ WM, recurring copy number alterations are rare in $MYD88^{WT}$ WM, including loss of chromosome 6q.

GENE EXPRESSION PROFILING

Transcriptome studies have allowed gene expression analysis based on underlying somatic gene mutations. Comparison of MYD88-mutated WM and healthy donor (HD) B cells showed increased expression of the VDJ recombination genes DNTT, RAG1, and RAG2, BCL2, as well as CXCR4 pathway genes.[42] The latter support a role for CXCR4 signaling regardless of underlying CXCR4 mutation status. Based on expression and pathway analysis studies, modulation of MYD88 signaling in context of CXCR4 mutations associated with the downregulation of TLR4, and increased transcription of IRAK3, the IRAK4/IRAK1 inhibitor. WM cells derived from patients with MYD88 WT also showed overexpression of DNTT, RAG1, RAG2, CXCL12, and VCAM1, but not BCL2 in distinction to MYD88-mutated disease. The latter may be clinically significant because the BCL2 inhibitor venetoclax is active in WM, although the importance of MYD88 mutation status remains to be clarified and may provide a biological marker for its use in WM.[43] Gene set enrichment analysis also indicated a downregulation of NFKB-induced TNFA signaling in patients with MYD88 WT relative to patients with MYD88-mutated WM, and an increase in AKT/mammalian target of rapamycin (MTOR) signaling. The latter is of clinical interest for exploration of PI3K or MTOR inhibitors in MYD88 WT WM.

SUMMARY

Next-generation sequencing has revealed recurring somatic mutations in WM that include MYD88, as well as CXCR4, ARID1A, and CD79B that typically accompany MYD88-mutated disease. In contrast, the genomic landscape of MYD88 WT WM includes mutations in many genes that are found in DLBCL, and include NFKB activating mutations that are downstream of BTK, as well as mutations in chromatin-modifying genes and DNA damage repair that are found in MYD88 WT disease. The genomic findings provide important insights into the pathogenesis, prognostication, and therapeutic development for WM.

REFERENCES

1. Hunter ZR, Yang G, Xu L, et al. Genomics, signaling, and treatment of Waldenström macroglobulinemia. J Clin Oncol 2017;35(9):994–1001.
2. Treon SP, Gustine J, Xu L, et al. MYD88 wild-type Waldenstrom macroglobulinaemia: differential diagnosis, risk of histological transformation, and overall survival. Br J Haematol 2018;180(3):374–80.
3. Hunter ZR, Tsakmaklis N, Demos M, et al. The genomic landscape of MYD88 wild-type Waldenström's macroglobulinemia is characterized by somatic mutations in TBL1XR1, the CBM complex, and NFKB2 [abstract: 4011]. Blood 2017;130.
4. Treon SP, Xu L, Yang G, et al. MYD88 L265P somatic mutation in Waldenstrom's macroglobulinemia. N Engl J Med 2012;367:826–33.
5. Xu L, Hunter Z, Yang G, et al. MYD88 L265P in Waldenstrom macroglobulinemia, immunoglobulin M monoclonal gammopathy, and other B-cell lymphoproliferative disorders using conventional and quantitative allele-specific polymerase chain reaction. Blood 2013;121:2051–8.
6. Varettoni M, Arcaini L, Zibellini S, et al. Prevalence and clinical significance of the MYD88 L265P somatic mutation in Waldenstrom macroglobulinemia, and related lymphoid neoplasms. Blood 2013;121:2522–8.
7. Jiménez C, Sebastián E, Del Carmen Chillón M, et al. MYD88 L265P is a marker highly characteristic of, but not restricted to, Waldenström's macroglobulinemia. Leukemia 2013;27:1722–8.
8. Poulain S, Roumier C, Decambron A, et al. MYD88 L265P mutation in Waldenstrom's macroglobulinemia. Blood 2013;121:4504–11.
9. Ansell SM, Hodge LS, Secreto FJ, et al. Activation of TAK1 by MYD88 L265P drives malignant B-cell growth in Non-Hodgkin lymphoma. Blood Cancer J 2014;4:e183.
10. Varettoni M, Zibellini S, Arcaini L, et al. MYD88 (L265P) mutation is an independent risk factor for progression in patients with IgM monoclonal gammopathy of undetermined significance. Blood 2013;122(13):2284–5.
11. Xu L, Hunter ZR, Yang G, et al. Detection of MYD88 L265P in peripheral blood of patients with Waldenström's Macroglobulinemia and IgM monoclonal gammopathy of undetermined significance. Leukemia 2014;28(8):1698–704.
12. Poulain S, Boyle EM, Roumier C, et al. MYD88 L265P mutation contributes to the diagnosis of Bing Neel syndrome. Br J Haematol 2014;167(4):506–13.
13. Gustine JN, Meid K, Hunter ZR, et al. MYD88 mutations can be used to identify malignant pleural effusions in Waldenström macroglobulinaemia. Br J Haematol 2018;180(4):578–81.
14. Tsakmaklis N, Xu L, Manning R, et al. Mutated MYD88 homozygosity is increased in previously treated patients with Waldenstrom's macroglobulinemia, and

associates with CXCR4 mutation status and ibrutinib exposure [abstract: 1462]. Blood 2017;130.

15. Treon SP, Xu L, Hunter ZR. MYD88 mutations and response to ibrutinib in Waldenström's macroglobulinemia. N Engl J Med 2015;373:584–6.

16. Lin SC, Lo YC, Wu H. Helical assembly in the MyD88-IRAK4-IRAK2 complex in TLR/IL-1R signalling. Nature 2010;465:885–90.

17. Ngo VN, Young RM, Schmitz R, et al. Oncogenically active MYD88 mutations in human lymphoma. Nature 2011;470:115–9.

18. Yang G, Zhou Y, Liu X, et al. A mutation in MYD88 (L265P) supports the survival of lymphoplasmacytic cells by activation of Bruton tyrosine kinase in Waldenström macroglobulinemia. Blood 2013;88:1222–32.

19. Liu X, Hunter ZR, Xu L, et al. Targeting myddosome assembly in Waldenstrom macroglobulinaemia. Br J Haematol 2017;177(5):808–13.

20. Yang G, Buhrlage S, Tan L, et al. HCK is a survival determinant transactivated by mutated MYD88, and a direct target of ibrutinib. Blood 2016;127:3237–52.

21. Schmidt J, Federmann B, Schindler J, et al. MYD88 L265P and CXCR4 mutations in lymphoplasmacytic lymphoma identify cases with high disease activity. Br J Haematol 2015;169:795–803.

22. Xu L, Hunter ZR, Tsakmaklis N, et al. Clonal architecture of CXCR4 WHIM-like mutations in Waldenström macroglobulinaemia. Br J Haematol 2016;172:735–44.

23. Poulain S, Roumier C, Venet-Caillault A, et al. Genomic landscape of CXCR4 mutations in Waldenstrom macroglobulinemia. Clin Cancer Res 2016;22:1480–8.

24. Hernandez PA, Gorlin RJ, Lukens JN, et al. Mutations in the chemokine receptor gene CXCR4 are associated with WHIM syndrome, a combined immunodeficiency disease. Nat Genet 2003;34:70–4.

25. Liu Q, Chen H, Ojode T, et al. WHIM syndrome caused by a single amino acid substitution in the carboxy-tail of chemokine receptor CXCR4. Blood 2012;120: 181–9.

26. Cao Y, Hunter ZR, Liu X, et al. CXCR4 WHIM-like frameshift and nonsense mutations promote ibrutinib resistance but do not supplant MYD88(L265P) -directed survival signalling in Waldenström macroglobulinaemia cells. Br J Haematol 2015;168:701–7.

27. Guerrera ML, Tsakmaklis N, Xu L, et al. MYD88 mutated and wild-type Waldenströms macroglobulinemia: characterization of chromosome 6q gene losses and their mutual exclusivity with mutations in CXCR4. Haematologica 2018. https://doi.org/10.3324/haematol.2018.190181.

28. Treon SP, Cao Y, Xu L, et al. Somatic mutations in MYD88 and CXCR4 are determinants of clinical presentation and overall survival in Waldenstrom's macroglobulinemia. Blood 2014;123:2791–6.

29. Cao Y, Hunter ZR, Liu X, et al. The WHIM-like CXCR4(S338X) somatic mutation activates AKT and ERK, and promotes resistance to ibrutinib and other agents used in the treatment of Waldenstrom's macroglobulinemia. Leukemia 2014;29: 169–76.

30. Roccaro AM, Sacco A, Jimenez C, et al. C1013G/CXCR4 acts as a driver mutation of tumor progression and modulator of drug resistance in lymphoplasmacytic lymphoma. Blood 2014;123:4120–31.

31. Wiegand KC, Shah SP, Al-Agha OM, et al. *ARID1A* mutations in endometriosis-associated ovarian carcinomas. N Engl J Med 2010;363:1532–43.

32. Guan B, Wang T-L, Shih I-M. ARID1A, a factor that promotes formation of SWI/SNF-mediated chromatin remodeling, is a tumor suppressor in gynecologic cancers. Cancer Res 2011;71:6718–27.

33. Seda V, Mraz M. B-cell receptor signaling and its crosstalk with other pathways in normal and malignant cells. Eur J Haematol 2015;94:193–205.
34. Wilson WH, Young RM, Schmitz R, et al. Targeting B cell receptor signaling with ibrutinib in diffuse large B cell lymphoma. Nat Med 2015;21:922–6.
35. Argyropoulos KV, Vogel R, Ziegler C, et al. Clonal B-cells in Waldenström's macroglobulinemia exhibit functional features of chronic active B-cell receptor signaling. Leukemia 2016;30:1116–25.
36. Chan VWF, Lowell CA, DeFranco AL. Defective negative regulation of antigen receptor signaling in Lyn-deficient B lymphocytes. Curr Biol 1998;8:545–53.
37. Jimenez C, Prieto-Conde I, García-Álvarez M, et al. Genetic characterization of Waldenstrom macroglobulinemia by next generation sequencing: an analysis of fourteen genes in a series of 61 patients [abstract: 2971]. Blood 2015;126.
38. Alonso S, Jimenez C, Alcoceba M, et al. Whole-exome sequencing of Waldenstrom macroglobulinemia transformation into aggressive lymphoma [abstract: 4101]. Blood 2016;128.
39. Schmitz R, Wright GW, Huang DW, et al. Genetics and pathogenesis of diffuse large B-cell lymphoma. N Engl J Med 2018;378(15):1396–407.
40. Chapuy B, Stewart C, Dunford AJ, et al. Molecular subtypes of diffuse large B cell lymphoma are associated with distinct pathogenic mechanisms and outcomes. Nat Med 2018;24(5):679–90.
41. Hunter ZR, Xu L, Yang G, et al. The genomic landscape of Waldenstrom macroglobulinemia is characterized by highly recurring MYD88 and WHIM-like CXCR4 mutations, and small somatic deletions associated with B-cell lymphomagenesis. Blood 2014;123(11):1637–46.
42. Hunter ZR, Xu L, Yang G, et al. Transcriptome sequencing reveals a profile that corresponds to genomic variants in Waldenström macroglobulinemia. Blood 2016;128:827–38.
43. Castillo JC, Gustine J, Meid K, et al. Prospective phase II study of venetoclax in patients with previously treated Waldenstrom macroglobulinemia [abstract: S854]. Proc Eur Hematol Assoc 2018.

Working Toward a Genomic Prognostic Classification of Waldenström Macroglobulinemia
C-X-C Chemokine Receptor Type 4 Mutation and Beyond

Marion Magierowicz, Pharm D[a], Cécile Tomowiak, MD[b],
Xavier Leleu, MD, PhD[b], Stéphanie Poulain, Pharm D, PhD[a,c,*]

KEYWORDS

- Waldenström macroglobulinemia • Next generation sequencing • *CXCR4* mutation
- *TP53* mutation • *CD79B* mutation

KEY POINTS

- CXCR4 mutations in the C terminal domain of CXCR4 have been identified in nearly one-third of patients with Waldenström macroglobulinemia.
- *CXCR4* mutations may have a prognostic impact, as identifying potential mechanisms of resistance to targeted drugs.
- Other variants in B-cell receptor or nuclear factor-κB pathways have been described at a lower frequency, and may play a key role either for prognostication or to better understand the Waldenström macroglobulinemia pathogenesis.
- Subclassification of Waldenström macroglobulinemia may consider integrating mutational profile.

INTRODUCTION

The *MYD88 L265P* mutation is the first described in Waldenström macroglobulinemia (WM),[1] and is a gain-of-function mutation present in more than 90% of patients with WM.[2] MYD88 is an adaptor protein that bridges Toll-like receptor (TLR) signaling

Part of the work referenced herein was supported by the Comité du Septentrion de la Ligue contre le Cancer and the Fondation Française pour la Recherche contre le Myélome et les Gammapathies (FFRMG).
Conflicts of Interests: No conflict of interest.
[a] Laboratory of Hematology, Biology and Pathology Center, CHU of Lille, Lille, France;
[b] Department of Hematology, Hospital of the Miletrie, INSERM CIC 1402, CHU of Poitiers, Poitiers, France; [c] INSERM UMR S 1172, Team 4, Cancer Research Institute, Lille, France
* Corresponding author. Laboratory of Hematology, Biology and Pathology Center, CHU of Lille, Lille, France.
E-mail address: stephanie.poulain@chru-lille.fr

Hematol Oncol Clin N Am 32 (2018) 753–763
https://doi.org/10.1016/j.hoc.2018.05.007
0889-8588/18/© 2018 Elsevier Inc. All rights reserved.

hemonc.theclinics.com

and the activation of canonical nuclear factor kappa B (NF-κB) signaling pathways.[3] Furthermore, whole-genome sequencing has also revealed others mutations in WM with various incidence rates, although significantly lower than *MYD88* mutation.[4] C-X-C chemokine receptor type 4 (*CXCR4*) mutations are the second most frequent somatic mutations, identified in approximately 30% of cases.[4,5]

Significant progress has been made in understanding the pathogenesis of this disease with the advent of next-generation sequencing (NGS).[6] WM has become a new model of a unifying single-hit lymphoid malignancy, with *MYD88* mutation being the driver event, and other mutation playing more of a prognostic or chemoresistance role. The goal of this review is to summarize our current knowledge of the mutational landscape of MW.

THE C-X-C CHEMOKINE RECEPTOR TYPE 12/ C-X-C CHEMOKINE RECEPTOR TYPE 4 AXIS IN WALDENSTRÖM MACROGLOBULINEMIA

CXCR4 is a G-protein–coupled receptor that plays an important role in normal lymphopoiesis and cell trafficking, particularly involved into homing to the bone marrow, along with its ligand, the stromal cell-derived factor-1 (CXCL12/SDF-1).[7] The CXCL12/CXCR4 axis promotes activation of several pathways including RAS, Akt, and NF-κB and interplays with the B-cell receptor (BCR) pathway.[8] CXCR4 is expressed by WM tumor cells, although the level of expression is similar to normal B cells in the bone marrow.[5,9] However, WM cells have increased expression of the CXCR4 ligand, CXCL12.[9,10] CXCR4 directly interacts with CD49 d in response to CXCL12 signaling in regulating migration and adhesion of WM cells to the bone marrow microenvironment. Inhibition of CXCR4 by plerixafor (AMD3100) abrogates transendothelial migration of WM cells and inhibits adhesion of WM cells to fibronectin.[9] The distal amino acid region of the C-terminus is known to regulate the signaling of CXCR4 by CXCL12. This domain plays a critical role in the desensitization process that contributes to the regulation of the signal transduction and CXCR4 expression.[8] Therefore, alteration of this domain might deregulate the CXCR4/SDF1 axis signaling pathway.[8]

C-X-C CHEMOKINE RECEPTOR TYPE 4 MUTATIONS

Up to one-third of patients with WM display a *CXCR4* mutation in the C-terminal domain, using different techniques. Allele-specific polymerase chain reaction, Sanger sequencing, or NGS were used to detect *CXCR4* mutations in selected as well as not tumoral cells (**Table 1**). *CXCR4* mutations (CXCR4^{Mut}) comprise more than 40 different point mutations, all targeting the 45 amino acid intracytoplasmic carboxy (C)-terminal tail, the inhibitory domain of CXCR4.[5,11–16] The mutation results in truncation of the CXCR4 protein leading to amplified CXCR4 mediated signaling. Two types of *CXCR4* mutations have been observed in nearly equal proportions in WM: the frame shift mutation (CXCR4^{FS}) and nonsense mutation types (CXCR4^{NS}). The CXCR4 S338X is a hotspot variant.[11] In WM primary cells, there was a significantly greater expression of CXCR4 protein in WM with *CXCR4* mutation, independent of the type of mutation.[5,11] All mutations were heterozygous, and no acquired uniparental disomy (loss of heterozygosity without variation of copy number) was observed at the *CXCR4* locus or variation of copy gene number (gain or deletion).[5] *CXCR4* mutations are rarely observed in marginal zone lymphoma, multiple myeloma, or chronic lymphocytic leukemia.[11,17–20] *CXCR4* mutations have been identified in rare diffuse large B-cell lymphoma cases.[21] Overall, *CXCR4* mutation is a new feature of WM.

Table 1
CXCR4 mutation spectrum in WM

	WM (No. of Patients)	Assay	*CXCR4* Mutation (%)	*CXCR4* C1013 A Mutation (%)	*CXCR4* Mutated Patients Characteristics
Treon et al,[12] 2014	175	Sanger sequencing on B selected cells	29	8	49% *CXCR4* nonsense mutation 51% *CXCR4* frameshift mutation Nonsense mutation had higher levels of bone marrow disease, higher serum IgM level, more frequent hyperviscosity syndrome No prognostic value on overall survival
Roccaro et al,[11] 2014	117	Q PCR C1013G		30	Not evaluated
Xu et al,[15] 2016	164	Sanger sequencing on B selected cells + Q PCR	39.6		43% not treated WM 34% of treated WM
Schmidt et al,[16] 2015	47	Sanger sequencing on bone marrow biopsy	36	14.8	Higher IgM monoclonal component, lower hemoglobin level, higher bone marrow infiltration
Ballester et al,[47] 2016	14	Sanger sequencing/ pyrosequencing	29	2/8	Not evaluated
Poulain et al,[25] 2017	98	NGS + Sanger sequencing on B selected cells	27	5	Thrombopenia, higher IgM monoclonal component
Baer et al,[48] 2017	78	NGS	25	12.8	Not evaluated
Jiménez et al,[14] 2018	54	NGS on CD19 selected cells + Q PCR	37		Higher IgM monoclonal component

Abbreviations: NGS, next-generation sequencing; Q PCR, real time polymerase chain reaction; WM, Waldenström macroglobulinemia.

C-X-C CHEMOKINE RECEPTOR TYPE 4 WHIM SYNDROME–LIKE MUTATIONS

Interestingly, somatic *CXCR4* mutations observed in tumor cells in WM are similar to a germline mutation found in the WHIM syndrome. This syndrome is a rare disease characterized by *w*arts, *h*ypogammaglobulinemia, recurrent *i*nfections, and bone marrow *m*yelokathexis resulting in chronic neutropenia.[22] This combined primary immunodeficiency disorder is caused by autosomal-dominant gain-of-function mutations in the C-terminal domain of CXCR4 receptor.[22,23] It is the only Mendelian condition related to mutation of a chemokine receptor.[22,23]

GENOMIC LANDSCAPE OF C-X-C CHEMOKINE RECEPTOR TYPE 4 MUTATIONS

The genomic landscape of *CXCR4* mutated WM was deciphered using a single nucleotide polymorphism array.[5] $CXCR4^{mut}$ had a greater frequency of genomic aberrations in WM compared with CXCR4[wild type], a particular feature associated with symptomatic WM or genomic instablity.[24,25] $CXCR4^{mut}$ had a greater incidence rate of trisomy 4, a greater frequency of gain of Xq, and of deletion 8p and 6q. Transcriptome sequencing reveals a profile that corresponds to genomic mutations of *MYD88* and *CXCR4* genes in WM.[26] *CXCR4* mutation identified a transcriptional signature characterized by downregulation of TLR4 signaling and activation of TLR7 pathway. MYD88 L265P and *CXCR4* mutations lead to initiate a cascade of downstream consequences individualizing 3 biological and clinical phenotypes.

C-X-C CHEMOKINE RECEPTOR TYPE 4 MUTATIONS AND WALDENSTRÖM MACROGLOBULINEMIA PATHOGENESIS

Approximately 10% to 20% of individuals with monoclonal gammopathy of undetermined significance (MGUS) have the IgM subtype associated with an increased risk of developing WM or other lymphoid malignancies.[27] Like with the *MYD88* mutation, *CXCR4* mutations may be an early event IgM MGUS, a premalignant status.[11–14,20] For instance, *CXCR4* C1013G mutation was identified in 8 of 40 individuals (20%) with IgM MGUS.[11] Targeted NGS of a series of 57 MGUS identified CXCR4 in 9% of cases.[13] However, the role of *CXCR4* mutation in transformation from MGUS to WM or to diffuse large B-cell lymphoma is not known.[28]

C-X-C CHEMOKINE RECEPTOR TYPE 4 MUTATION IMPACTS WALDENSTRÖM MACROGLOBULINEMIA TUMOR CELL BEHAVIOR

Recent studies have characterized the functional relevance of the CXCR4[C1013G] somatic variant, demonstrating that it acts as an activating mutation, responsible for enhanced WM cell dissemination leading to extramedullary localization and disease progression in vivo.[11] *CXCR4*-mutated WM cells present with an enrichment for mRNAs related to oncogenesis, cell proliferation, tumor invasiveness, and antiapoptosis, further confirming the activating role of the $CXCR4^{C1013G}$ variant in WM. Preclinical studies with the most common *CXCR4 S338X* mutation in WM have shown sustained signaling of AKT, ERK, and BTK after CXCL12 binding in comparison with wild-type *CXCR4*, as well increased cell growth and survival of WM cells.[11] A WHIM mutation in the G-protein–coupled receptor, CXCR4, results in the permanent activation by its ligand, CXCL-12 leading to activation of AKT1 and mitogen-activated protein kinase, as well as migration, adhesion, and homing of WM cells to the bone marrow niches, thereby promoting survival. Direct inhibition of *MYD88* L265P signaling overcomes CXCL12-trigered survival effects in *CXCR4* mutated cells, supporting a primary role for MYD88 signaling in WM.[29] One might propose that the type of mutation does not matter much in WM, in contrast with the loss of C-terminus domain of CXCR4 protein, in which modified function might play a role in WM pathogenesis.

C-X-C CHEMOKINE RECEPTOR TYPE 4 MUTATION, A DRIVER OF DRUG RESISTANCE

CXCR4 mutations mediate drug resistance to mammalian target of rapamycin, PI3K, and BTK inhibitors by blocking CXCR4 receptor internalization and leading to a persistently activated CXCR4 that in turn prolongs and enhances activation of AKT1 and mitogen-activated protein kinase, an alternative pathway that may contribute to resistance to BTK inhibition independent of the *CXCR4* mutation type.[29,30] Importantly,

CXCR4-mutated cells also presented increased resistance to ibrutinib treatment in vitro.[11,30] In preclinical observations, venetoclax, a first-in-class BCL2 selective inhibitor, seems to induce direct apoptosis and enhance ibrutinib and idelalisib-triggered apoptosis, irrespective of the CXCR4 mutation status, providing a rationale for investigating this promising drug as monotherapy or combination approaches.[31] Venetoclax synergistically enhances the antiproliferative effects of ibrutinib and overcomes ibrutinib resitance.[32] The role of CXCR4 mutation in ibrutinib resistance were also validated in the clinical setting, in patients with WM enrolled in the ibrutinib clinical trial.[33]

C-X-C CHEMOKINE RECEPTOR TYPE 4 MUTATION IS ASSOCIATED WITH A PARTICULAR CLINICAL PRESENTATION

From a clinical standpoint, WM with CXCR4 mutation had a specific clinicobiological profile associated with features characterized by more aggressive disease features and adverse prognosis in WM. Overall, CXCR4 mutations have been associated with lower leukocyte, hemoglobin, and platelet counts; higher serum IgM levels related to greater marrow involvement; higher International Prognostic Scoring System for Waldenström Macroglobulinemia score with adverse features; and more symptomatic disease requiring therapy.[12] There seems to be a greater risk of developing hyperviscosity syndrome requiring therapy.[12,34] The association to thrombocytopenia was described in most studies.[5,12,16] Phenotypically, such patients were less likely to have adenopathy.[12]

C-X-C CHEMOKINE RECEPTOR TYPE 4 MUTATION AND PROGNOSIS

The question of CXCR4 mutation prognostic value is still debated in WM. Despite difference in clinical presentation, CXCR4 mutation do not seem to adversely affect overall survival in retrospective studies.[5,12,13] The prognostic value of CXCR4 mutation may be questioned according to the treatment schema as suggesting by in vitro resistance in CXCR4-mutated models. BTK inhibition has become an important therapeutic approach in WM as primary therapy and also in relapsed/refractory WM. CXCR4 mutation was associated with lower response rates to ibrutinib and delayed responses. CXCR4 mutations were independently associated with a 4-fold increased odds of ibrutinib discontinuation.[34] Mutation of BTK C481S associated with ibrutinib resistance may cooccur in patients with CXCR4 mutatations.[35] The responses of second-generation proteasome inhibitor, carfilzomib, were achieved irrespective of the MYD88 and CXCR4 status.[36] Further studies are needed to explore the prognosis value of CXCR4 mutation in WM in large clinical trials.

Alteration of B-Cell Receptors in Waldenström Macroglobulinemia

WM clonal B cells exhibit functional features of chronic active BCR signaling, a pathway regulated by CD79B, CD79A, and LYN.[37] In WM, LYN copy number loss is observed in nearly 60% of cases and may favor alteration of BCR response.[6] CD79B is somatically mutated in nearly 10% of cases of WM,[5,12–14] with a hotspot on tyrosine residues 196 (Y196), corresponding with the immunoreceptor tyrosine-based activation motif that is essential to transmitting BCR signaling.[38] Comparatively, CD79A mutations are less frequent.[39] Although not yet demonstrated in WM, CD79A and CD79B mutations are important to identify because they have been reported to be associated with resistance to BCR inhibitors in MYD88 mutated diffuse large B-cell lymphoma.[40] Furthermore, CD79B mutation was recently described as a potential driver of diffuse large B-cell lymphoma transformation of WM. CARD11 mutations are rare but emergence of *CARD11* mutated clone may be observed in ibrutinib-resistant WM.[5,35]

Mutation in DNA Repair Pathway and Chromatin Remodeling

TP53 is a tumor suppressor gene mapped at the chromosome 17p13 locus that functions as a regulator of cellular response to DNA damage.[41] Combining Sanger sequencing, NGS, and single nucleotide polymorphism array studies, several patterns of TP53 alteration were observed in WM: monoallelic loss, mutations, or acquired uniparental disomy. TP53 alteration is identified in nearly 10% of patients with WM, of whom two-thirds are mutated in the DNA-binding domain.[4,25] TP53 mutations are highly correlated with deletion of 17p and complex genomic features suggesting a greater genomic instability. Patients with WM with a TP53 mutation more often had poor outcome in WM, independent of International Prognostic Scoring System for Waldenström Macroglobulinemia score or CXCR4 or MYD88 L265P mutations.[25]

AT-rich interactive domain 1A (*ARID1A*) is a key component of the switch/sucrose nonfermentable chromatin remodeling complex that uses the energy of adenosine triphosphate hydrolysis to remodel chromatin structure.[42] *ARID1a* mutation was described in up to 17% of WM.[6,13,14] Most variants were frameshift mutation or missense variants leading to loss of function of ARID1a. WM with *ARID1a* mutation had greater bone marrow disease involvement and lower hemoglobin and platelet counts.[4] No prognostic value of these variants is reported to date.[6]

MLL2 is a histone methyltransferase that participates in the methylation of Lys-4 of histone H3. Although initially described in 2 patients with *MYD88* wild-type WM,[12] *MLL2* mutations was then reported on a higher incidence, up to 22%, also in MYD88 L265P mutated WM.[13]

Nuclear Factor-κB Pathway Mutation

A high frequency of copy number alteration of NF-κB pathway family gene was described in WM in addition to *MYD88* mutation[39,43] (**Fig. 1**). Deletion of 6q is one of the most frequent abnormalities in WM arising in 20% to 40% of cases.[24,39,44] Inactivation of negative regulators of NF-κB signaling pathways by mutation has been shown in WM. The study of minimal deleted regions in 6q has highlighted the potential role of *TNFAIP3*, a tumor suppressor gene. In WM, homozygous inactivating mutation at *TNFAIP3* is a rare event (<5% of cases).[4,45] In contrast, monoallelic deletions of 6q, including *TNFAIP3*, is more frequently observed in nearly 30% of WM and was associated with lower TNFAIP3 transcript expression levels.[45] This finding may suggest *TNFAIP3* haploinsufficiency in WM. In contrast, proliferation and NF-κB activation induced by MYD88L265P were nevertheless rapidly countered by the induction of TNFAIP3, supporting the role of alteration of NF-κB inhibitors in the regulation of constitutive activation of master pathways in WM.[46] *TRAF3* encodes a putative ubiquitin ligase. Constitutive activation of the noncanonical pathway is a consequence of TRAF3 inactivation by mutation. Although not unique to WM, biallelic inactivation of *TRAF3* is recurrent findings in a small percentage (<5%) of patients with WM.[4,13,45]

Genomic Classification for Waldenström Macroglobulinemia

There have been a number of studies describing in detail the genomic alterations in WM, including single nucleotide polymorphism array, comparative genomic hybridization, and whole exome sequencing, and whole genome sequencing. The next question is, therefore, whether it is time to propose a new pathogenesis-based classification of WM, whether these genomic abnormalities dictate the prognosis and/or mechanisms

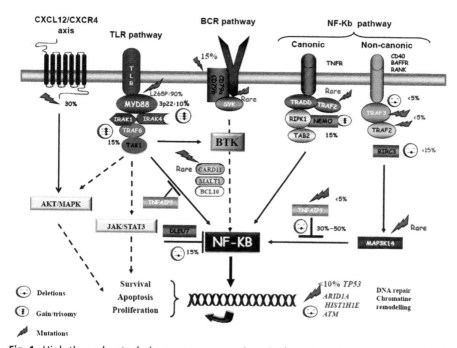

Fig. 1. High-throughput whole-genome sequencing, single nucleotide polymorphism (SNP), and comparative genomic hybridization (CGH) array have identified several pathways characterized with recurrent genomic alterations in Waldenström macroglobulinemia (WM). Several mechanisms of action are involved in the gene deregulation of key signaling pathways, including deletion, mutation, acquired uniparental disomy (UPD), and gain of chromosome. A constitutive activation of nuclear factor-κB (NF-κB) was demonstrated in WM cells. Genes of canonical and noncanonical NF-κB pathways, CXCR4, Toll-like receptors (TLR), and B-cell receptor (BCR) may be activated deregulation of survival, apoptosis and proliferation, which may lead to WM clone expansion and tumor progression. (*Adapted from* Poulain S, Herbaux C, Bertrand E, et al. Genomic studies have identified multiple mechanisms of genetic changes in Waldenström Macroglobulinemia. Clin Lymphoma Myeloma Leuk 2013;13(2):203; with permission.)

of resistance to drugs, and, finally, whether the mutational landscape may actually dictate therapeutic options.

The composite molecular architecture in WM has been mapped out. The *CXCR4*-mutated cases simultaneously harbor *MYD88* mutations in most cases.[4,5] BCR mutations seem to be mutually exclusive to *CXCR4* in *MYD88 L265P* mutated WM.[5] The molecular landscape of *CXCR4* mutation in WM showed existence of intraclonal (variation in coexpression of *MYD88* and *CXCR4* mutations) and interclonal (*BCR* and *CXCR4* mutations in MYD88 L265P WM) heterogeneity. Overall, these data may suggest the following hypothesis: where *MYD88* L265P mutation is a founder mutation in WM, a first genetic hit that would promote NF-κB and JAK-STAT3 signaling.[3] From a mechanistic hypothesis, a complex rather than a unique deregulation of the TLR/NF-κB pathway characterizes *MYD88* L265P WM with other interconnected pathways or alterations of copy number or other regulators of this pathway (**Fig. 2**). Therefore, *MYD88* mutation has become a diagnostic tool and an important event in WM pathogenesis.[1,2] Subclonal mutation of *CXCR4* may suggest a later event during disease course because they are subclonal in nearly one-third of patients with WM.[5,15,31] As

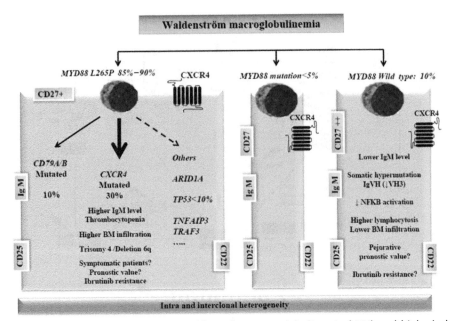

Fig. 2. Mutational classification in Waldenström macroglobulinemia (WM) and biological relevance to clinical presentation. MYD88L265P is mutated in nearly 90% of cases. Other *MYD88* mutations are now described. *CXCR4* mutation is mainly observed in MYD88L265P mutated WM. Although CXCR4 is expressed in all subgroups, the 3 genotypes correspond with 3 different signatures of transcriptional profiling or clonal. BM, bone marrow.

described in others lymphoid malignancy, this subclonal process may be not limited to passenger mutations, but is observed in driver mutations, such as *MYD88* or *CXCR4*.[17,18] In contrast, mutations in DNA repair such as *TP53* mutations are independent of *CXCR4* or *MYD88* mutations, suggesting different genetic interaction according to the type of pathway[25] (see **Fig. 2**). CXCR4 and *TP53* mutations are more related to prognostication either direct prognosis or indirect by development of mechanisms of resistance.

Importantly, these data plead for studying the mutational landscape of WM, at least *MYD88* mutation for diagnosis, *TP53* mutations for direct prognostication, and *CXCR4* and *TP53* mutations to tailor therapy inducing mechanisms of resistance to BTK and BCR/PI3K pathways-based inhibitors.[1,33] Interestingly, BTK inhibitors may induce in vitro apoptosis and loss of viability in WM, independent of p53 alteration in cell lines and primary WM cells, and may suggest that BTK inhibitors may be an interesting therapeutic option to *TP53* alteration WM, similar to chronic lymphocytic leukemia.[17,25] The ability to overcome these potential mechanisms of resistance by using combinations of drugs is unknown. Taking together, these data favor a first mutational-based algorithm in WM.

SUMMARY

The past 5 years have brought a tremendous amount of data to WM to better understand the various aspects of the disease pathogenesis, prognostication, and even understanding potential mechanisms of resistance to drugs. This disease is now a new oncogenic model with MYD88 L265P as a key driver genetic determinant. Other mutations such as *CXCR4* may modulate the clonal evolution in conjunction with copy number variation or epigenetic abnormalities. Some datasets have further outlined the genomic heterogeneity of WM and, subsequently, the existence of genetic interaction beyond the current indolent versus symptomatic classification. Finally, ongoing studies will help to decipher the clonal longitudinal evolution of WM; therefore, providing a better way of understanding the mutational landscape at relapse, given that WM remains a disease that systematically evolves toward relapse. Ultimately, this knowledge will translate into practical therapeutic application(s), although how this application will emerge remains a challenge in the near future. One of the greatest aspects of this concept of genomically driven algorithm for the treatment of WM comes to develop novel chemotherapy-free options.

REFERENCES

1. Castillo JJ, Garcia-Sanz R, Hatjiharissi E, et al. Recommendations for the diagnosis and initial evaluation of patients with Waldenström Macroglobulinaemia: a Task Force from the 8th International Workshop on Waldenström Macroglobulinaemia. Br J Haematol 2016;175:77–86.
2. Treon SP, Xu L, Yang G, et al. MYD88 L265P somatic mutation in Waldenström's Macroglobulinemia. N Engl J Med 2012;367:826–33.
3. Jeelall YS, Horikawa K. Oncogenic MYD88 mutation drives Toll pathway to lymphoma. Immunol Cell Biol 2011;89:659–60.
4. Hunter ZR, Xu L, Yang G, et al. The genomic landscape of Waldenström macroglobulinemia is characterized by highly recurring MYD88 and WHIM-like CXCR4 mutations, and small somatic deletions associated with B-cell lymphomagenesis. Blood 2014;123:1637–46.
5. Poulain S, Roumier C, Caillault-Venet A, et al. Genomic landscape of CXCR4 mutations in Waldenström Macroglobulinemia. Clin Cancer Res 2016;22:1480–8.
6. Hunter ZR, Ynag G, Xu L, et al. Genomics, signaling, and treatment of Waldenström macroglobulinemia. J Clin Oncol 2017;35:994–1001.
7. Burger JA, Gribben JG. The microenvironment in chronic lymphocytic leukemia (CLL) and other B cell malignancies: insight into disease biology and new targeted therapies. Semin Cancer Biol 2014;24:71–81.
8. Scala S. Molecular pathways: targeting the CXCR4–CXCL12 axis—untapped potential in the tumor microenvironment. Clin Cancer Res 2015;21:4278–85.
9. Ngo HT, Leleu X, Lee J, et al. SDF-1/CXCR4 and VLA-4 interaction regulates homing in Waldenstrom macroglobulinemia. Blood 2008;112:150–8.
10. Poulain S, Ertault M, Leleu X, et al. SDF1/CXCL12 (-801GA) polymorphism is a prognostic factor after treatment initiation in Waldenstrom macroglobulinemia. Leuk Res 2009;33:1204–7.
11. Roccaro A, Sacco A, Jimenez C, et al. C1013G/CXCR4 acts as a driver mutation of tumor progression and modulator of drug resistance in lymphoplasmacytic lymphoma. Blood 2014;123:4120–31.
12. Treon SP, Cao Y, Xu L, et al. Somatic mutations in MYD88 and CXCR4 are determinants of clinical presentation and overall survival in Waldenstrom macroglobulinemia. Blood 2014;123:2791–6.
13. Varettoni M, Zibellini S, Defranscesco I, et al. Pattern of somatic mutations in patients with Waldenström macroglobulinemia or IgM monoclonal gammopathy of undetermined significance. Haematologica 2017;102:2077–85.

14. Jiménez C, Prieto-Conde M, Garcia-Alvarez M, et al. Unraveling the heterogeneity of IgM monoclonal gammopathies: a gene mutational and gene expression study. Ann Hematol 2018;97:475–84.
15. Xu L, Hunter Z, Tsakmaklis N, et al. Clonal architecture of CXCR4 WHIM-like mutations in Waldenström Macroglobulinaemia. Br J Haematol 2016;172:735–44.
16. Schmidt J, Federmann B, Schindler N, et al. MYD88 L265P and CXCR4 mutations in lymphoplasmacytic lymphoma identify cases with high disease activity. Br J Haematol 2015;169:795–803.
17. Lazarian G, Guièze R, Wu CJ. Clinical implications of novel genomic discoveries in chronic lymphocytic leukemia. J Clin Oncol 2017;35:984–93.
18. Walker BA, Boyle EM, Wardell CP, et al. Mutational spectrum, copy number changes, and outcome: results of a sequencing study of patients with newly diagnosed myeloma. J Clin Oncol 2015;33:3911–20.
19. Spina V, Rossi D. Molecular pathogenesis of splenic and nodal marginal zone lymphoma. Best Pract Res Clin Haematol 2017;30:5–12.
20. Cao X, Meng Q, Cai H, et al. Detection of MYD88 L265P and WHIM-like CXCR4 mutation in patients with IgM monoclonal gammopathy related disease. Ann Hematol 2017;96:971–6.
21. Reddy A, Zhang J, Davis N, et al. Genetic and functional drivers of diffuse large B cell lymphoma. Cell 2017;171:481–94.
22. Al Ustwani O, Kurzrock R, Wetzler M. Genetics on a WHIM. Br J Haematol 2014; 164:15–23.
23. Hernandez PA, Gorlin R, Lukens J, et al. Mutations in the chemokine receptor gene CXCR4 are associated with WHIM syndrome, a combined immunodeficiency disease. Nat Genet 2003;34:70–4.
24. Poulain S, Roumier C, Galiegue-Zouitina S, et al. Genome wide SNP array identified multiple mechanisms of genetic changes in Waldenstrom macroglobulinemia. Am J Hematol 2013;88:948–54.
25. Poulain S, Roumier C, Bertrand E, et al. TP53 mutation and its prognostic significance in Waldenstrom's macroglobulinemia. Clin Cancer Res 2017;23:6325–35.
26. Hunter ZR, Xu L, Yang G, et al. Transcriptome sequencing reveals a profile that corresponds to genomic variants in Waldenström macroglobulinemia. Blood 2016;128:827–38.
27. Mailankody S, Landgren O. Monoclonal gammopathy of undetermined significance and Waldenström's macroglobulinemia. Best Pract Res Clin Haematol 2016;29:187–93.
28. Jiménez C, Alonso-Alvarez S, Alcoceba M, et al. From Waldenström's macroglobulinemia to aggressive diffuse large B-cell lymphoma: a whole-exome analysis of abnormalities leading to transformation. Blood Cancer J 2017;7:e591.
29. Cao Y, Hunter Z, Liu X, et al. CXCR4 WHIM-like frameshift and nonsense mutations promote ibrutinib resistance but do not supplant MYD88L265P-directed survival signalling in Waldenström macroglobulinaemia cells. Br J Haematol 2015; 168:701–7.
30. Cao Y, Hunter Z, Liu X, et al. The WHIM-like CXCR4S338X somatic mutation activates AKT and ERK and promotes resistance to ibrutinib and other agents used in the treatment of Waldenstrom's Macroglobulinemia. Leukemia 2015;29:169–76.
31. Cao Y, Ynag G, Hunter Z, et al. The BCL2 antagonist ABT-199 triggers apoptosis, and augments ibrutinib and idelalisib mediated cytotoxicity in CXCR4 Wild-type and CXCR4 WHIM mutated Waldenstrom macroglobulinaemia cells. Br J Haematol 2015;170:134–8.

32. Paulus A, Akhtar S, Yousaf H, et al. Waldenstrom macroglobulinemia cells devoid of BTKC481S or CXCR4WHIM-like mutations acquire resistance to ibrutinib through upregulation of Bcl-2 and AKT resulting in vulnerability towards veneto-clax or MK2206 treatment. Blood Cancer J 2017;7:e565.

33. Treon SP, Tripsas C, Meid K, et al. Ibrutinib in previously treated Waldenström's macroglobulinemia. N Engl J Med 2015;372:1430–40.

34. Gustine JN, Meid K, Dubeau T, et al. Ibrutinib discontinuation in Waldenström macroglobulinemia: etiologies, outcomes, and IgM rebound. Am J Hematol 2018;93(4):511–7.

35. Xu L, Tsakmaklis N, Yang G, et al. Acquired mutations associated with ibrutinib resistance in Waldenström macroglobulinemia. Blood 2017;129:2519–25.

36. Treon SP, Tripsas C, Meid K, et al. Carfilzomib, rituximab, and dexamethasone (CaRD) treatment offers a neuropathy-sparing approach for treating Waldenström's macroglobulinemia. Blood 2014;124:503–10.

37. Argyropoulos KV, Vogel R, Ziegler C, et al. Clonal B cells in Waldenström's macroglobulinemia exhibit functional features of chronic active B-cell receptor signaling. Leukemia 2016;30:1116–25.

38. Davis RE, Ngo V, Lenz G, et al. Chronic active B-cell-receptor signalling in diffuse large B-cell lymphoma. Nature 2010;463:88–92.

39. Poulain S, Roumier C, Herbaux C, et al. Genome wide SNP Array (SNPa) analysis reveals clonal evolution during clinical course in Waldenstrom's Macroglobulinemia (WM). Blood 2012;120:297.

40. Wilson WH, Young R, Schmitz R, et al. Targeting B cell receptor signaling with ibrutinib in diffuse large B cell lymphoma. Nat Med 2015;21:922–6.

41. Muller PA, Vousden KH. Mutant p53 in cancer: new functions and therapeutic opportunities. Cancer Cell 2014;25:304–17.

42. Wu R, Wang T, Shih IM. The emerging roles of ARID1A in tumor suppression. Cancer Biol Ther 2014;15:655–64.

43. Poulain S, Roumier C, Decambron A, et al. MYD88 L265P mutation in Waldenstrom macroglobulinemia. Blood 2013;121:4504–11.

44. Nguyen-Khac F, Lambert J, Chapiro E, et al. Chromosomal aberrations and their prognostic value in a series of 174 untreated patients with Waldenström's macroglobulinemia. Haematologica 2013;98:649–54.

45. Braggio E, Keats JJ, Leleu X, et al. Identification of copy number abnormalities and inactivating mutations in two negative regulators of nuclear factor-κB signaling pathways in Waldenström's macroglobulinemia. Cancer Res 2009;69:3579–88.

46. Wang JQ, Jeelall YS, Beutler B, et al. Consequences of the recurrent MYD88L265P somatic mutation for B cell tolerance. J Exp Med 2014;211:413–26.

47. Ballester LY, Loghavi S, Kanagal-Shamanna R, et al. Clinical validation of a CXCR4 mutation screening assay for Waldenstrom macroglobulinemia. Clin Lymphoma Myeloma Leuk 2016;16:395–403.

48. Baer C, Dicker F, Kern W, et al. Genetic characterization of MYD88-mutated lymphoplasmacytic lymphoma in comparison with MYD88-mutated chronic lymphocytic leukemia. Leukemia 2017;31:1355–62.

Flow Cytometry

Amaia Gascue, BSª, Juana Merino, MD, PhDª, Bruno Paiva, PhDª,b,c,d,*

KEYWORDS

- Waldenström macroglobulinemia • Flow cytometry • Immunophenotyping • B cells
- Plasma cells

KEY POINTS

- The Waldenström's clone (B cells and plasma cells) harbors unique immunophenotypic characteristics that differ from other gammopathies and immunoglobulin M (IgM)–secreting lymphomas.
- IgM monoclonal gammopathy of undetermined significance and smoldering WM display clonal B cells with the phenotypic signature of the malignant WM clone.
- Multiparameter flow cytometry (MFC) immunophenotyping identifies high-risk smoldering WM and symptomatic WM patients with inferior outcomes.
- Response assessment by MFC is highly predictive of progression-free and overall survival.

INTRODUCTION

The World Health Organization defines Waldenström macroglobulinemia (WM) as a lymphoplasmacytic lymphoma (LPL) associated with a monoclonal immunoglobulin M (IgM) protein, and bone marrow (BM) infiltration by small lymphocytes that may exhibit plasma cell (PC) differentiation.[1] Because LPL infrequently involves the lymph nodes or other extramedullary sites, demonstration of BM infiltration (eg, through trephine biopsy) is therefore essential for the diagnosis of WM.[2] Many patients who fulfill the criteria for WM do not require immediate therapy because they are detected before developing disease-related symptoms.[3] These patients are classified as smoldering WM, a clinically recognized entity with a cumulative probability of progression to symptomatic WM, amyloidosis, or lymphoma of 65% at 10 years.[4] Smoldering WM

Disclosure Statement: All authors declared no conflicts of interest.
This study was supported by the International Waldenström Macroglobulinemia Foundation and the Leukemia & Lymphoma Society (IWMF/LLS) Strategic Research Roadmap Initiative (MACRO-NEXT).
ª Department of immunology, Clínica Universidad de Navarra, Av. Pio XII, 36, Pamplona, 31008, Spain; b Centre for Applied Medical Research (CIMA), Pamplona, Spain; c Healthcare Research Institute of Navarre (IDISNA), Pamplona, Spain; d CIBERONC, Spain
* Corresponding author. Centre for Applied Medical Research (CIMA), Av. Pio XII 55, Pamplona 31008, Spain.
E-mail address: bpaiva@unav.es

patients have a greater risk of progression to full-blown disease than IgM monoclonal gammopathy of undetermined significance (MGUS) cases (18% at 10 years).[5] There is some controversy to distinguish between smoldering WM and IgM MGUS; some groups use the amount of serum concentration of the M-protein and BM infiltration, whereas a consensus panel defined BM disease involvement on histologic examination as the main criterion.[2,6] It is plausible to assume that similarly to multiple myeloma (MM), most (if not all) WM patients have eventually gone through the benign stages of IgM MGUS and smoldering WM before developing clinical symptoms.[7] Therefore, the availability of objective criteria for the differential diagnosis between these conditions as well as more accurate estimation of their risk of progression is important to individualize monitoring of patients with premalignant conditions.

Multiparameter flow cytometry (MFC) immunophenotyping has been a mainstay in the diagnosis and monitoring of most hematologic malignancies.[8–12] Together, with the patient's clinical history, analytical results, and morphologic assessment of blood and marrow smears, MFC is also part of the initial diagnostic workup, mainly because of its ability to typically provide conclusive results within a few hours. It should be noted that MFC immunophenotyping provides accurate assessment of the expression of multiple markers and their fluorescence intensity in thousands of individual cells, and allows clear discrimination between aberrant and both normal and reactive cells, even when they are present at low or very low frequencies in a sample.[13] These are unique features of MFC because conventional morphologic approaches fail to distinguish clonal from normal cells, and molecular approaches mainly focus on the detection of specific genetic markers in whole BM and not in single cells.[13] Thus, a growing number of studies have applied MFC immunophenotyping to the study of IgM MGUS or WM (**Fig. 1**), and its utility will be reviewed here.

THE IMMUNOPHENOTYPIC ATLAS OF THE NORMAL B-CELL DEVELOPMENT

The origin of B-cell malignancies is associated with three main stages of B-cell differentiation:

i. B-lymphoblastic leukemias/lymphomas arise during the development of naive B cells from hematopoietic stem cells in the BM;
ii. B-cell lymphoproliferative disorders have been associated with antigen-dependent differentiation of naive B cells into memory B cells in secondary lymphoid tissues (lymph nodes and mucosa-associated lymphoid tissues), BM, and spleen; and

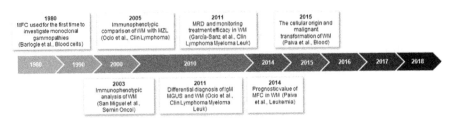

Fig. 1. Time axis highlighting the most important discoveries concerning MFC and its use in WM. (*Modified from* Jelinek T, Bezdekova R, Zatopkova M, et al. Current applications of multiparameter flow cytometry in plasma cell disorders. Blood Cancer J 2017;7(10):e617; with permission.)

iii. Monoclonal gammopathies arise from PCs that, most frequently, accumulate in the BM.

Thus, precise knowledge about the normal B-cell differentiation contributes to understanding the classification of B-cell neoplasms and, subsequently, to more specific and sensitive diagnosis (**Fig. 2**).[14,15]

Naive B cells with mature phenotypic characteristics (CD20[+] CD19[+] CD38low[+] CD27[−] coexpression) of surface membrane (sm) IgM and smIgD leave the BM to enter the peripheral blood and recirculate. When naive B cells encounter their cognate antigen in the lymph nodes presented by follicular dendritic cells and interact with antigen-specific T cells, they become activated and form a germinal center under the regulation of BCL6. In the germinal center, cells undergo rapid proliferation, somatic hypermutation of the immunoglobulin heavy (IGH) chain variable regions, IGH isotype class switch recombination, and an increment in BCR affinity for the antigen (affinity maturation).[15]

Upregulation of CD10, CD38, CD95, and HLA-DR and decreased CD44 and BCL2 expression discriminate germinal center B cells from other B-cell subsets in the lymph nodes (ie, naive, memory B cells, and plasmablasts). In contrast to germinal center B cells, memory B cells have increased levels of IL-2 receptors (CD25) and Fas (CD95) proapoptotic molecules, and decreased expression of CD23 and CD200.[16] Half of memory B cells in peripheral blood have undergone Ig class switch recombination, and the other half still coexpresses surface IgM and IgD, or IgM alone. Some investigators have observed that smIgM[+] smIgD[+] memory B cells have undergone less proliferation than germinal center cells, with a lower median number of somatic hypermutations than switched memory B cells. On the other hand, this population contains cells with the same phenotypic characteristics and IGHV gene repertoire as germinal-center–derived smIgG memory B cells. These apparently controversial observations may indicate that the sIgM[+] sIgD[+] subset comprises a mixture of germinal center and nongerminal center memory B cells.[15]

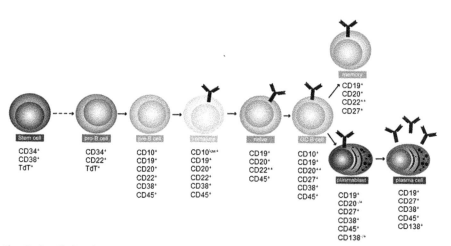

Fig. 2. B-cell development. The diagram describes the phenotype of B cells at different stages of maturation. (*Modified from* Perez-Andres M, Paiva B, Nieto WG, et al. Human peripheral blood B-cell compartments: a crossroad in B-cell traffic. Cytometry B Clin Cytom 2010;78 Suppl 1:S56; with permission.)

Afterward, B cells develop to PCs and search for survival niches in the BM or mucosa-associated lymphoid tissues to complete their differentiation to long-life antibody-secreting PCs. The former show stronger positivity for CD27 than memory B cells, together with high expression of CD38 and lack CD25. Most normal BM PCs are CD19+, CD45dim, CD56−, and CD81+, but some are CD19−, CD45−, CD56+, or CD81−, in multiple possible combinations.[17,18] PCs in peripheral blood seem to comprise a heterogeneous pool of cells from different tissues and with different degrees of maturation. Accordingly, these show phenotypic features of new-born plasmablasts from secondary lymphoid tissues (smIgH+ CD20+ HLA-DR+) and PCs that are phenotypically closer to their mature BM counterpart (eg, lack of the previous markers, together with expression of CD138); however, PCs displaying phenotypes that fully overlap with that of plasmablasts or BM PCs are not detectable in peripheral blood, and some markers are exclusively expressed in the corresponding tissue (eg, CD10 by secondary lymphoid tissue plasmablasts and CD56 in BM PCs).[15,16,19,20]

THE WALDENSTRÖM MACROGLOBULINEMIA B-CELL CLONE AND ITS NORMAL COUNTERPART

According to their phenotypic and molecular profile, WM has been associated with antigen-driven differentiation. Clonal lymphocytes in WM are characterized by the surface expression of pan B cell markers (CD19, CD20, CD22) and monoclonal expression of smIgM restricted to kappa or lambda light chain expression (**Fig. 3A**).[21,22] A summary of immunophenotypic differences between normal and neoplastic WM cells are shown in **Table 1**. In comparison with normal mature B cells, CD22 expression in WM is lower, whereas there are no significant changes in the levels of expression of CD19, CD20, and the B-cell receptor. CD25 is expressed homogenously in malignant WM cells (**Fig. 4A**). In contrast to hairy cell leukemia, WM cells are usually negative for CD103 and CD11c. Expression of CD10, typically associated with germinal center B cells, is most frequently negative in WM. Although half of WM cases express CD38, their expression is lower than progenitor B cells and PCs. The memory-surrogate marker CD27 displays heterogenous expression, from negative to dim and bright reactivity (**Fig. 4B**). Clonal B cells are positive for CD79b, CD81, CD24, HLA-DR, and BCL2 in a high proportion of cases. CD5, CD23, and CD200 could be detected in a smaller fraction of WM patients (CD5 and CD23 in <20% and CD200 in 60% of the patients).[23,24] CD305 (LAIR1) is usually

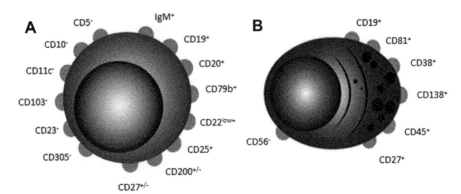

Fig. 3. Immunophenotype of the WM clone: (*A*) B cells and (*B*) PCs.

Table 1
Differences between Waldenström macroglobulinemia clone, memory B cell, and marginal zone lymphoma

Antigen	Memory B Cell	WM B Cell	MZL
CD5	−	−	−
CD10	−	−	−
CD11C	−	−	+/−
CD19	++	++	++
CD20	++	++	++
CD22	+	Low+	Low+
CD23	−	+/−	+/−
CD25	−/+	+	+/−
CD27	+/−	+/−	−
CD38	−/+	−/+	−/+
CD305	+/−	−	+
SIG	+	+	+

Antigen expression: +, positive; ++, intense positive; −, negative; −/+, heterogeneous negative to positive.

negative, which contrasts to its heterogenous expression on normal B cells. Morever, there is a monoclonal expression of surface immunoglobulins light chain with a predominance of kappa versus lambda (κ:λ ratio of 5:1).[25]

Taken together, the most common immunophenotype of WM clonal B cells could be described as follows: CD19$^+$, CD22^{low+}, CD20$^+$, CD25$^+$, CD27$^{+/-}$, CD5$^-$, CD10$^-$, CD11c$^-$, and CD38$^{-/+}$. Therefore, considering this immunophenotype, the origin of WM cells could be placed as postgerminal center cells that have been activated.[15] Furthermore, clonotypic cells are seen within the lymphoid and PC compartments implying a certain degree of differentiation.[26]

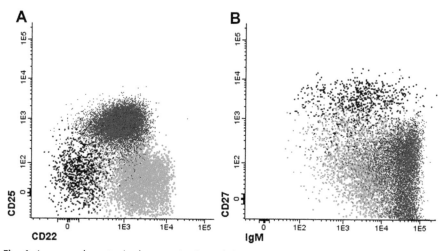

Fig. 4. Immunophenotypic characterization of the WM clone. (*A, B*) WM B-cell clone (*red*), WM PC clone (*blue*), and mature normal B cells (*green*) dot-blot for CD25 versus CD22 and CD27 versus surface IgM, respectively.

THE WALDENSTRÖM MACROGLOBULINEMIA PLASMA CELL CLONE AND ITS NORMAL COUNTERPART

The phenotype of PCs in patients with IgM MGUS and WM is very similar to that of normal PC (**Fig. 3**B).[27] Most WM PCs do not express pan B-cell markers such as CD20 or CD22, lack smIg, and share the same clonal cytoplasmic staining of light chains (ie, cyKappa or cyLambda) as WM B cells. As compared with their normal counterpart, PCs show variable yet mostly positive expression of CD19, CD27, CD45, and CD81.[17,18] It should be noted that in 40% of patients with WM it is possible to identify a clear population of plasmablasts (**Fig. 5**); these cells are defined by strong expression of CD19, CD27, CD45, and CD38, partial reactivity for CD138, together with progressive downregulation of CD20.[20]

DIAGNOSTIC UTILITY OF MULTIPARAMETER FLOW CYTOMETRY IMMUNOPHENOTYPING
Differential Diagnosis

Already more than 10 years ago, the Second International Workshop on WM agreed in that the diagnosis of WM should be supported by immunophenotypic studies.[2] Some immunophenotypic and morphologic features of WM show significant overlap with marginal zone lymphoma (MZL), and accordingly, this is one of the most challenging differential diagnoses (**Fig. 6**; see **Table 1**).[28] In fact, MZL could present with relatively monoclonal IgM and lymphoplasmacytic component infiltration in some patients. No clear differences between the antigenic profiles of WM and MZL have been reported.[29,30] Both express pan B markers (CD19, CD20, CD22), but their expression (particularly CD22 expression) is weaker in WM than in MZL. SmIgM expression is higher in WM than MZL, and there is a marked predominance of kappa versus lambda in WM, whereas in patients with MZL, kappa and lambda relation is similar. CD5, CD23, CD103, and CD10 are negative in both diseases. CD11c could contribute to

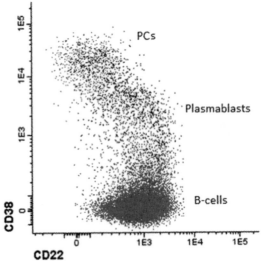

Fig. 5. The WM clone represented by a continuum of small B cells, plasmablasts, and PCs. The WM clone represented by a continuum of small B cells (*red*), plasmablasts (*black*), and PCs (*blue*).

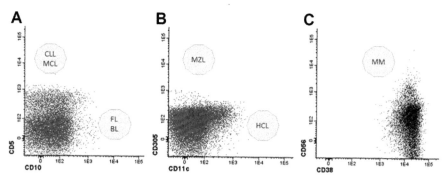

Fig. 6. WM's B-cell (*red*) and PC clone (*blue*) immunophenotype. (*A–C*) CD5, CD10, CD305, CD11c, CD38, and CD56 versus a schematic representation of the typical phenotype present in B-cell CLL, MCL, FL, Burkitt lymphoma (BL), MZL, hairy cell leukemia (HCL), and MM.

distinguish WM from MZL because it is positive in 33% of WM compared with the 70% of MZL.[29] CD25 along with CD305 are other markers that can help to distinguish both entities. CD25 is expressed in most patients with WM, whereas only in a half of patients with MZL. CD305 is upregulated in MZL, whereas in WM it is usually negative. Other 2 markers that help discriminating between WM and MZL are sIgM and CD79b, which are overexpressed in WM.[25] Another difference between WM and MZL is the increased numbers of mast cells seen in the former.[21]

Other IgM-secreting lymphoproliferative disorders, such as mantle cell lymphoma (MCL), follicular lymphoma (FL), or chronic lymphocytic leukemia (CLL), should also be considered in the differential diagnosis of WM (see **Table 1**).[24] On immunophenotypic grounds, CD5 and CD23 expression are used to support the diagnosis of CLL, whereas expression of CD5 in the absence of CD23 would suggest the diagnosis of MCL. Dim or partial expression of CD5 and/or CD23 may be seen, however, in WM. In such cases, CLL could be excluded based on bright surface immunoglobulin light chain and bright CD20 expression. Other relevant markers to distinguish WM from CLL are sIgM and CD79b that are downregulated in CLL.[25] FL with BM involvement and IgM paraprotein could be differentiated from WM because CD10 is typically expressed in FL.

As noted above, the phenotype of WM PCs overlaps with that of normal PCs and, accordingly, clearly differs from that of MM patients (**Table 2**). Compared with WM,

Table 2
Differences between Waldenström macroglobulinemia plasma cell, normal, and multiple myeloma's plasma cell

Antigen	Normal PC	WM PC	MM PC
CD19	+	+	− (96%)
CD20	−	+ (30%)	−/+ (17%)
CD27	++	+	− or −/+ (68%)
CD45	+	+	− (80%)
CD56	−	−	+ (60%)
CD81	+	+	−/+
CD117	−	−	+ (32%)

Antigen expression: +, positive; ++, intense positive; −, negative; −/+, heterogeneous negative to positive; in parentheses: frequency of antigen pattern.

MM PCs can be identified by MFC based on 3 major characteristics: underexpression of CD19, CD27, CD38, CD45, and CD81; overexpression of CD28, CD33, CD56, CD117, and CD200; and asynchronous expression of CD20 and smIg. When compared with MM, PCs from WM patients show higher expression of CD19 and CD45.[17,31] Moreover, WM PC are smaller than MM PC based on forward scatter.

Once the diagnosis of other entities has been excluded, patients must be staged into IgM-MGUS, smoldering or symptomatic WM.[27] Similarly to MM, also in WM there may be a continuum between IgM MGUS and WM, rather than these entities being considered as separate. MFC shows a continuously evolving immunophenotypic pattern from IgM-MGUS to smoldering and symptomatic WM. Such phenotypic profile is consistent with a progressive accumulation of light-chain restricted mature B cells up to the stage of a lymphoplasmacytic cell, which shows a characteristic Waldenström's phenotype: SmIgM+/CD22low+/CD25+.[27] However, further investigations with the input of novel polychromatic cytometry and multidimensional analysis of flow cytometry data were warranted to elucidate if reveiled that the phenotypic differences between IgM MGUS and WM patients as regards the B-cell compartment are related to the expansion of the WM clone from one stage to the other. Accordingly, recent findings denoted a common phenotypic signature for IgM MGUS and WM, suggesting a common cellular origin (ie, CD25+ CD22low+ activated B-lymphocytes) and a potential unifying genetic event (eg, MYD88 L265P) rendering the WM signature.

IgM MGUS and WM are typically different in the percentage of BM infiltration by B cells.[26] Different cutoffs of B-lymphocyte infiltration have been used to differentiate between IgM MGUS and WM (smoldering and symptomatic), ranging from 10% to 30%.[26] These results slightly differ from cutoffs established by the Mayo Clinic, which recommended at least 10% infiltration as a threshold to distinguish IgM MGUS from WM.[32] According to the Spanish experience using MFC, the median percentage of mature BM B cells (among total nucleated cells) progressively increases ($P<.001$) from IgM MGUS (2.2%) to smoldering (8.7%) and symptomatic WM patients (12.2%). In fact, only 1% of IgM MGUS patients showed greater than 10% B cells, in contrast to 34% and 55% of smoldering and symptomatic WM patients ($P<.001$). As could be expected, this was associated with a progressively increased ($P<.001$) infiltration by light-chain-isotype–positive B cells (as reflected by the percentage of B cells with cytoplasmic expression of the patient-specific light-chain isotype within the mature B-cell compartment) from IgM MGUS to smoldering and symptomatic WM patients (median of 75%, 96%, and 99%, respectively). Consequently, only 1% of IgM MGUS patients showed full light-chain restriction of the B-cell compartment (as reflected by the absence of B cells with cytoplasmic expression of the uninvolved light chain), in contrast to 19% and 40% of smoldering and symptomatic WM patients ($P<.001$). Despite similar percentages of BM PCs (among total nucleated cells) are found among IgM MGUS and WM patients, a progressively higher degree of light-chain-isotype–positive PCs (as reflected by the percentage of PCs with cytoplasmic expression of the patient-specific light-chain isotype within the PC compartment) was also noted from IgM MGUS to smoldering to symptomatic WM: median of 70%, 85%, and 97%, respectively. Although such findings could be potentially attributed to peripheral blood contamination of BM specimens or due to specific PC loss during sample preparation, it could also reflect an intrinsic feature of WM biology; in fact, increasing numbers of BM PCs are typically detected by MFC in MM as compared with MGUS patients. Taken together, current data support a potential value of MFC immunophenotyping for the differential diagnosis of IgM MGUS versus WM.

Prognostic Value

MFC is a valuable technique to assess the tumor burden and the degree of clonality in patients' BM aspirate. A retrospective study on 244 newly diagnosed patients (67, IgM MGUS; 77, smoldering WM; and 100 symptomatic WM) revealed that BM B cells progressively increased from IgM MGUS to smoldering WM and symptomatic WM patients.[27] The increase of B lymphocytes is accompanied by an increase of infiltration by light-chain–restricted B cells. Smoldering WM patients who had BM infiltration with more than 10% of B cells and full light chain restriction of the B-cell compartment had higher risk of progression into symptomatic WM. Moreover, in symptomatic WM patients with less than 10% B cells and retaining normal mature B cells, a more indolent disease was observed with prolonged overall survival as compared with other patients. By contrast, the analyses of the PC compartment afford no prognostic value.

MONITORING OF THE WALDENSTRÖM MACROGLOBULINEMIA CLONE

At present, BM evaluation is only performed to confirm CR, which requires the absence of malignant cells by morphologic evaluation. However, it is becoming clear that there is not a perfect correlation between the immunoglobulin responses and BM response. IgM responses are slow with purine analogue and monoclonal antibody-based therapy (eg, through anti-CD20) because these agents selectively deplete B cells but not PCs. Therefore, the complete eradication of clonal B cells but not PCs may translate into a favorable outcome despite suboptimal response according to current criteria (that is, persistent M protein).[33] This discrepancy has led to a reevaluation of the value of BM assessments.[34] Recently, it has been suggested the determination of MYD88 mutational status as predictive data for treatment response in WM. However, a recent retrospective study revealed that MYD88 L265P is present in both clonal B cells and PCs derived from individual WM patients.[35] Therefore, with the availability of more effective therapies for WM, it will be critical to combine sensitive and comprehensive monitoring of clonality in both B cells and PCs together with the evaluation of serum M protein. Accordingly, these observations highlight MFC as a potential technique to assess response in WM.

García-Sanz and colleagues[36] evaluated the value of response assessment by MFC in the BM of 42 WM patients. The persistence of abnormal B cell was strongly associated with the depth of conventional response criteria, although there were some cases with small discordances (persistence of high number of tumor cells despite a partial response, or significant reduction of clonal B cells despite persistently high levels of serum monoclonal IgM protein). MFC resulted in a better predictor of survival than serum determinations. The data showed that less than 5% of abnormal B cells were associated with longer duration of response, progression-free survival, and overall survival. These results merit future investigations in prospective studies in order to assess if it can be used a surrogate marker for WM outcome and whether it could be of help to tailor the type and the length of the therapy in these patients.

SUMMARY

MFC plays a significant role during the differential diagnosis of IgM-secreting disorders, because this technique can provide relatively fast and conclusive results, helping to distinguish between reactive and malignant conditions as well as to help classify different monoclonal gammopathies and other lymphoproliferative disorders.

Currently, this technique is particularly useful to distinguish WM from other B-cell lymphoproliferative disorders and from related IgM monoclonal gammopathies based on the specific immunophenotype of WM B cells and PCs. In addition, MFC appears to be a valuable technique to assess response in WM.

REFERENCES

1. Swerdlow SH, Campo E, Harris NL, et al. WHO classification of tumours of haematopoietic and lymphoid tissues. 4th Edition. International Agency for Research on Cancer; 2008.

2. Owen RG, Treon SP, Al-Katib A, et al. Clinicopathological definition of Waldenström's macroglobulinemia: consensus panel recommendations from the Second International Workshop on Waldenström's macroglobulinemia. Semin Oncol 2003; 30(2):110–5.

3. Gertz MA. Waldenström macroglobulinemia: 2012 update on diagnosis, risk stratification, and management. Am J Hematol 2012;87(5):503–10.

4. Kyle RA, Benson JT, Larson DR, et al. Progression in smoldering Waldenstrom macroglobulinemia: long-term results. Blood 2012;119(19):4462–6.

5. Kyle RA, Therneau TM, Rajkumar SV, et al. Long-term follow-up of IgM monoclonal gammopathy of undetermined significance. Blood 2003;102(10):3759–64.

6. Kyle RA, Rajkumar SV. Criteria for diagnosis, staging, risk stratification and response assessment of multiple myeloma. Leukemia 2009;23(1):3–9.

7. Weiss BM, Abadie J, Verma P, et al. A monoclonal gammopathy precedes multiple myeloma in most patients. Blood 2009;113(22):5418–22.

8. Kaleem Z, Crawford E, Pathan MH, et al. Flow cytometric analysis of acute leukemias. Diagnostic utility and critical analysis of data. Arch Pathol Lab Med 2003; 127(1):42–8.

9. Braylan RC. Impact of flow cytometry on the diagnosis and characterization of lymphomas, chronic lymphoproliferative disorders and plasma cell neoplasias. Cytometry 2004;58A(1):57–61.

10. Kwok M, Rawstron AC, Varghese A, et al. Minimal residual disease is an independent predictor for 10-year survival in CLL. Blood 2016;128(24):2770–3.

11. Theunissen P, Mejstrikova E, Sedek L, et al. Standardized flow cytometry for highly sensitive MRD measurements in B-cell acute lymphoblastic leukemia. Blood 2017;129(3):347–57.

12. Grimwade D, Freeman SD. Defining minimal residual disease in acute myeloid leukemia: which platforms are ready for "prime time"? Hematology 2014; 2014(1):222–33.

13. Paiva B, Almeida J, Pérez-Andrés M, et al. Utility of flow cytometry immunophenotyping in multiple myeloma and other clonal plasma cell-related disorders. Cytometry B Clin Cytom 2010;78(4):239–52.

14. Cooper MD. The early history of B cells. Nat Rev Immunol 2015;15(3):191–7.

15. García-Sanz R, Jiménez C, Puig N, et al. Origin of Waldenstrom's macroglobulinaemia. Best Pract Res Clin Haematol 2016;29(2):136–47.

16. Perez-Andres M, Paiva B, Nieto WG, et al. Human peripheral blood B-cell compartments: a crossroad in B-cell traffic. Cytometry B Clin Cytom 2010;78(Suppl 1):S47–60.

17. Flores-Montero J, de Tute R, Paiva B, et al. Immunophenotype of normal vs. myeloma plasma cells: toward antibody panel specifications for MRD detection in multiple myeloma. Cytometry B Clin Cytom 2016;90(1):61–72.

18. Paiva B, Puig N, Cedena MT, et al. Differentiation stage of myeloma plasma cells: biological and clinical significance. Leukemia 2017;31(2):382–92.

19. Kjeldsen MK, Perez-Andres M, Schmitz A, et al. Multiparametric flow cytometry for identification and fluorescence activated cell sorting of five distinct B-Cell subpopulations in normal tonsil tissue. Am J Clin Pathol 2011;136(6):960–9.
20. Caraux A, Klein B, Paiva B, et al. Circulating human B and plasma cells. Age-associated changes in counts and detailed characterization of circulating normal CD138- and CD138+ plasma cells. Haematologica 2010;95(6):1016–20.
21. San Miguel JF, Vidriales MB, Ocio E, et al. Immunophenotypic analysis of Waldenstrom's macroglobulinemia. Semin Oncol 2003;30(2):187–95.
22. Morice WG, Chen D, Kurtin PJ, et al. Novel immunophenotypic features of marrow lymphoplasmacytic lymphoma and correlation with Waldenström's macroglobulinemia. Mod Pathol 2009;22(6):807–16.
23. Konoplev S, Medeiros LJ, Bueso-Ramos CE, et al. Immunophenotypic profile of lymphoplasmacytic lymphoma/Waldenström macroglobulinemia. Am J Clin Pathol 2005;124(3):414–20.
24. Hunter ZR, Branagan AR, Manning R, et al. CD5, CD10, and CD23 expression in Waldenstrom's macroglobulinemia. Clin Lymphoma 2005;5(4):246–9.
25. Paiva B, Corchete LA, Vidriales M-B, et al. The cellular origin and malignant transformation of Waldenstrom macroglobulinemia. Blood 2015;125(15):2370–80.
26. Ocio EM, del Carpio D, Caballero Á, et al. Differential diagnosis of IgM MGUS and WM according to B-lymphoid infiltration by morphology and flow cytometry. Clin Lymphoma Myeloma Leuk 2011;11(1):93–5.
27. Paiva B, Montes MC, García-Sanz R, et al. Multiparameter flow cytometry for the identification of the Waldenström's clone in IgM-MGUS and Waldenström's Macroglobulinemia: new criteria for differential diagnosis and risk stratification. Leukemia 2014;28(1):166–73.
28. Harmon CM, Smith LB. B-cell Non-Hodgkin Lymphomas with plasmacytic differentiation. Surg Pathol Clin 2016;9(1):11–28.
29. Ocio EM, Hernandez JM, Mateo G, et al. Immunophenotypic and cytogenetic comparison of Waldenstrom's macroglobulinemia with splenic marginal zone lymphoma. Clin Lymphoma 2005;5(4):241–5.
30. Thieblemont C, Felman P, Callet-Bauchu E, et al. Splenic marginal-zone lymphoma: a distinct clinical and pathological entity. Lancet Oncol 2003;4(2):95–103.
31. Paiva B, Merino J, San Miguel JF. Utility of flow cytometry studies in the management of patients with multiple myeloma. Curr Opin Oncol 2016;28(6):511–7.
32. Kyle RA, Benson J, Larson D, et al. IgM monoclonal gammopathy of undetermined significance and smoldering Waldenström's macroglobulinemia. Clin Lymphoma Myeloma 2009;9(1):17–8.
33. Jelinek T, Bezdekova R, Zatopkova M, et al. Current applications of multiparameter flow cytometry in plasma cell disorders. Blood Cancer J 2018;8(1):e621.
34. Owen RG, Kyle RA, Stone MJ, et al. Response assessment in Waldenström macroglobulinaemia: update from the VIth International Workshop. Br J Haematol 2013;160(2):171–6.
35. Gustine J, Meid K, Xu L, et al. To select or not to select? The role of B-cell selection in determining the *MYD88* mutation status in Waldenström macroglobulinaemia. Br J Haematol 2017;176(5):822–4.
36. García-Sanz R, Ocio E, Caballero A, et al. Post-treatment bone marrow residual disease > 5% by flow cytometry is highly predictive of short progression-free and overall survival in patients with Waldenström's macroglobulinemia. Clin Lymphoma Myeloma Leuk 2011;11(1):168–71.

The Bone Marrow Microenvironment in Waldenström Macroglobulinemia

Shahrzad Jalali, PhD, Stephen M. Ansell, MD, PhD*

KEYWORDS

- Waldenström macroglobulinemia • Bone marrow niche • Homing
- Microenvironment • Cytokines • Immune cells • Angiogenesis

KEY POINTS

- An endosteal niche and vascular niche in the bone marrow provide support for lympho-plasmacytic cells.
- CXCR4 expressing malignant B cells home to the bone marrow in response to SDF-1.
- Bone marrow cells, including mast cells, monocytes, T cells, and endothelial cells, promote a favorable environment for malignant cells in Waldenström macroglobulinemia.
- Cytokines, including CCL5, IL-6, IL-21, and CXCL13, promote malignant B-cell growth, and CXCL13 levels are associated with responses to BTK inhibitors.

INTRODUCTION

Waldenström macroglobulinemia (WM) is a rare low-grade B-cell lymphoproliferative disorder defined by infiltration of lymphoplasmacytic lymphoma in the bone marrow (BM) and an increase synthesis by malignant cells with subsequent accumulation in the serum of monoclonal immunoglobulin M (IgM) that can cause hyperviscosity and other symptoms in the affected patients.[1] Recently, substantial research has been focused on understanding the pathogenesis of WM and to define the underlying molecular mechanisms involved in the disease. This work has confirmed not only the importance of mutations within the malignant cells but also highlighted the role for the BM microenvironment in promoting malignant B-cell growth, tumor cell survival, and IgM production. Using whole-genome sequencing analysis, initial work identified a somatic variant in the Myeloid Differentiation factor 88 (*MYD88*) gene that results in an amino acid leucine substitution by proline (L256P), and this mutation is seen in the vast majority of patients with WM.[2]

MYD88 is integral in processing signals external to cell and acts as an adaptor protein for interleukin-1R (IL-1R) and Toll-Like receptor (TLR) signaling pathways. Recent

Conflict of Interest: The authors have no conflicts of interest.
Division of Hematology, Mayo Clinic, 200 First Street Southwest, Rochester, MN 55905, USA
* Corresponding author.
E-mail address: ansell.stephen@mayo.edu

Hematol Oncol Clin N Am 32 (2018) 777–786
https://doi.org/10.1016/j.hoc.2018.05.005
0889-8588/18/© 2018 Elsevier Inc. All rights reserved.

data have also shown a role for MYD88 in B-cell receptor signaling. Overall, its role is to recruit signaling molecules and kinases that ultimately converge in nuclear factor (NF)κB activation.[3] TLRs are involved in regulating the innate immune response, and stimulation of TLR, induced by environmental signals, recruits MYD88 to the cytoplasmic domain of TLR. It then forms a complex with IL-1R associated kinase 4 (IRAK4) and IRAK1 and initiates a signaling cascade that subsequently activates NFκB.[4] Bruton tyrosine kinase (BTK) is also a component of TLR signaling that specifically binds to MYD88 and activates signaling cascades in response to environmental signals.[5] In WM, the mutant form of *MYD88* is shown to form a complex with BTK and induces constitutive activation of TLR, which amplifies the signaling process, and results in increased survival and proliferation of the tumor cells.[6] In addition to promoting NFκB signaling, the *MYD88* mutation has been shown to trigger Janus kinase/Signal transducer and activator of transcription 3 (JAK/STAT3) signaling and promote the secretion of cytokines, including IL-6, IL-10, and interferon-β (IFN-β) in the BM microenvironment. The accumulation of these cytokines in the tumor microenvironment enhances the survival of malignant cells via an autocrine mechanism,[7,8] implying that the *MYD88* mutation not only dysregulates malignant cell growth, but also amplifies signals from the BM environment, thereby further promoting uncontrolled lymphoma cell growth and increased IgM production.

A number of recent studies have focused on understanding the role of the BM microenvironment in WM, and these studies are exploring the role of other nonmalignant cells, cytokines, and other growth factors in WM pathology. Studies have suggested a reciprocal interaction between WM cells and the elements of the BM and shown that this interaction provides a growth support for WM cells. In this review, the authors summarize data regarding the key elements in the BM microenvironment that support the growth of lymphoplasmacytic lymphoma cells and stimulate monoclonal IgM production.

COMPONENTS OF THE BONE MARROW NICHE

The physical environment surrounding the malignant cell is important, and the architecture of the BM milieu incorporates both cellular and noncellular components. A wide variety of cell types, including blood cells and their lineages, including fibroblasts, mesenchymal cells, osteoblasts, osteoclasts, adipocytes, and endothelial cells are present, as well as noncellular components, such as extracellular matrix, cytokines, chemokines, growth factors, and metabolites.[9,10] Various studies have shown that a complex, yet coordinated array of the interactions exists between the cellular and acellular entities of the BM microenvironment. These interactions are a key determinant of survival and self-renewal of the hematopoietic stem cells (HSCs) in the BM and also in the differentiation of various cell types under physiologic conditions.[9,10]

Previous research has shown that 2 distinct specialized microenvironments, described as an endosteal niche and a vascular niche, are present in the BM, and these niches are shown to provide support for HSCs. The endosteal niche is localized at the interface of the trabecular bone with the BM elements, where the HSCs are in close proximity to cells such as osteoblasts. These cells maintain the self-renewal capacity of the HSCs and regulate their function. Interaction of HSCs with osteoblasts is mediated either directly through cell-cell contact or indirectly via secretory factors that are produced by osteoblasts and bind to their cognate receptor on HSCs. The endosteal niche therefore plays an essential role in sustaining HSCs, thereby allowing them to maintain the self-renewal capacity of the BM. In contrast, the vascular niche supports HSCs that are located near sinusoidal blood vessel structures, and the vascular niche facilitates dissemination of cells into the vascular system and also promotes "homing" of circulating cells from blood back to the BM.[11,12] Although the BM is the primary site for normal hematopoiesis, it may become a permissive environment for the location and growth of malignant cells due to these favorable BM niches. BM infiltration is a commonly seen in WM, and BM involvement in WM is commonly in a paratrabecular pattern,[5,11,13] suggesting that the BM niche supports and even promotes malignant cell growth.

MOLECULES THAT REGULATE HOMING OF MALIGNANT CELLS TO THE BONE MARROW

Previous studies have investigated the mechanisms by which WM cells home to the BM. This work has shown that stromal derived factor-1 (SDF-1; also known as CXCL12) is highly expressed in the BM of patients with WM, and the presence of SDF-1 results in dose-dependent migration of WM cells in vitro. The SDF-1–induced migration by WM cells is mediated by C-X-C chemokine receptor type 4 (CXCR4) on the cell surface, and inhibition of CXCR4 by the small molecule inhibitor plerixafor or by knockdown techniques substantially reduces WM cell migration.[14] These findings are highly relevant, as approximately 30% of the patients with WM have somatic mutations in the CXCR4 gene, and this mutation is the second most prevalent somatic mutation in WM after mutations in MYD88.[7,8] Initial research studied the cell surface expression of mutant CXCR4 and found that mutant CXCR4 is highly expressed on WM cells. This study found that increased CXCR4 expression, together with increased SDF-1 levels in patients with WM, could augment the CXCR4/SDF-1 interaction and significantly promote homing of WM cells to the BM.[15] SDF-1 has also been shown to be involved in the adhesion of WM cells to the fibronectin. WM cells have increased expression of Very Late Antigen-4 (VLA-4), an integrin dimer that co-interacts with CXCR4 and mediates adhesion of WM cells to the BM stromal cells (BMSCs) and endothelial cells in response to SDF-1. Furthermore, adhesion of WM cells to stromal cells from the BM has been found to make WM cells resistant to chemotherapy, suggesting that stromal cells play an important role in drug resistance providing a potential opportunity to exploit this therapeutically.[14]

Furthermore, activation of survival signaling pathways impacts WM cell homing to the BM. Akt activity has been found to be constitutively upregulated in malignant WM cells. In vivo and in vitro studies have demonstrated that activation of Akt not only induces proliferation but also influences migration and homing of the WM cells to the BM.[16] MicroRNA (miRNA), including MiR-155, regulates Akt, and WM cells have altered miRNA expression profiles compared with their normal cellular counterparts. Using miRNA expression profiling, it has been found that several miRNAs including MiR-155 are upregulated in malignant WM cells. MiR-155 plays an important role in B-cell malignancies and regulates the BMSC-induced proliferation of WM cells, modulates the adhesion of WM to the fibronectin, and induces the migration of the cells in response to SDF-1, thereby resulting in homing of the WM cells in the BM.[17]

CELLS IN THE BONE MARROW THAT FACILITATE TUMOR CELL GROWTH

WM cells do not grow in isolation in the BM; instead, normal cells that typically facilitate hematopoiesis, immunity, and bone formation surround them. The BM typically consists of T cells (CD4$^+$, CD8$^+$, and T$_{reg}$ cells), B cells, dendritic cells, natural killer cells, myeloid-derived suppressor cells, mesenchymal stem cells, osteoclasts, osteoblasts, and endothelial cells. Although the number and/or function of these cells can vary under pathologic circumstances, the contribution of these cells to the pathogenesis of WM has not been fully evaluated. Recently, several studies have reported that mast cells, T cells, monocytes, and endothelial cells may contribute to the pathogenesis of WM (**Fig. 1**).

Mast Cells

Increased numbers of mast cells in the BM is a characteristic of WM. It has been demonstrated that the mast cells in the BM of patients with WM promote the proliferation of malignant cells, and this support of malignant growth is mediated by the interaction of CD154 (CD40 L) and CD40, which are expressed on mast cells and malignant cells, respectively.[18] Although the signaling mechanisms regulating cell surface expression of CD40 and CD40 L are not well understood, previous work has described a role for soluble CD27 (sCD27), a member of the tumor necrosis factor (TNF) family. These studies have found that sCD27 is increased in the serum of the patients with active WM and induces the expression of CD40 L on mast cells, thereby promoting the CD40-CD40 L interaction. Of note, increased sCD27 in WM correlates with the serum IgM level, implying that it could serve as a marker for disease progression.[19]

T Cells

T cells present in the BM of patients with WM are thought to possibly represent part of an antitumor immune response; however, expression of immune checkpoint molecules on the surface of T cells is associated with an exhausted T-cell phenotype and recent work has shown that immune checkpoint molecules are expressed in both normal and WM marrows. The expression of programmed death-1 (PD-1) and its ligands, PD-L1 and PD-L2, has been found to be increased in WM, and the increased expression of PD-L1 and PD-L2 in the BM of the patients with WM modulates the proliferation of both the malignant B cells and normal T cells.[20] These findings suggest that T cells present in the BM are inhibited by the expression of immune

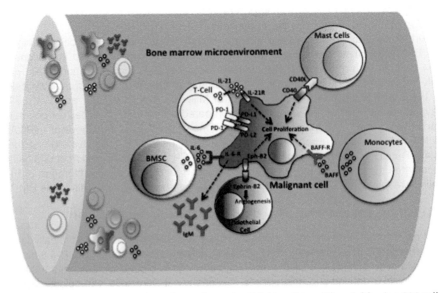

Fig. 1. Schematic representation of a malignant cell interacting with neighboring BM cells in WM.

checkpoint molecules on malignant cells and the PD-1/PD-1 ligand interactions may favor the growth and survival of the malignant clone.

Endothelial Cells

WM cells have also been shown to interact with endothelial cells in the BM microenvironment. Ephrin receptor-B2 (Eph-B2), a transmembrane receptor tyrosine kinase, is upregulated on WM cells, and its interaction with the ligand Ephrin-B2 on the endothelial cell surface induces WM cell adhesion and proliferation.[21] Co-culture of WM cells with endothelial cells promotes Eph-B2/EphrinB2 interaction and induces phosphorylation of Eph-B2, resulting in downstream signaling including activation of Akt, cyclin D3, cyclin E, focal adhesion kinase, Src, P130, paxillin, and cofilin. Activation of these molecules has been found to induce WM cell proliferation and adhesion. In contrast, downregulation of Eph-B2 on WM cells reduces the BM infiltration by malignant cells and inhibits tumor progression.[21]

CYTOKINES IN THE BONE MARROW MICROENVIRONMENT

Soluble factors, particularly cytokines, are critical regulators of B-cell differentiation to plasma cells and also facilitate plasma cell homeostasis and stimulate immunoglobulin secretion in the BM. For example, IL-21 is integral to the regulation of normal B-cell function and facilitates B-cell differentiation to immunoglobulin-producing plasma cells.[22] B-cell activating factor (BAFF), also known as B-lymphocyte stimulator (BLyS), is a member of the TNF superfamily that binds to its receptor on B cells (BAFF-R), promotes B-cell survival, and induces B-cell proliferation.[23] IL-6 also induces B-cell differentiation, stimulates immunoglobulin production, and promotes plasma cell survival.[24,25] Although cytokines are required to maintain normal B-cell function, dysregulation of their production or function will result in increased malignant cell growth.

A comprehensive analysis of the cytokine composition of the BM microenvironment in patients with WM found that it is very different from that of normal BM.[26] Using a multiplex bead-based array analysis to screen the cytokine expression in healthy controls and patients with WM, cytokines including chemokine (C-C Motif) ligand 5 (CCL5), granulocyte colony-stimulating factor (G-CSF), soluble IL-2 receptor (sIL-2R), epidermal growth factor, and IL-8 were found to be most different in their expression, with CCL5 showing the greatest increase in the patients with WM as compared with healthy subjects.[27] In this study, increased expression of CCL5 in the BM of patients with WM correlated with high IgM secretion and increased infiltration of the BM by malignant cells. To understand the function of CCL5 and define its potential role in modulating the BM microenvironment in WM, further research found that CCL5 does not directly impact the survival, growth rate, or IgM secretion in malignant WM cells. Rather, CCL5 indirectly modulates WM cell function by stimulating BMSCs to secrete IL-6 and the increased secretion of IL-6 stimulates WM cells to secrete IgM by a mechanism that involves JAK/STAT signaling.[27] The role of IL-6 in promoting IgM secretion also involves GLI2, an oncogenic zinc finger transcription factor, which is expressed in the BM of patients with WM. GLI2 induces transcription and cell surface expression of IL-6 receptor-α (IL-6Rα) on WM cells and promotes IgM secretion.[28] All told, increased expression of both IL-6 and IL-6Rα result in increased IgM secretion.

Similarly, IL-21 plays an important role in promoting WM cell growth and survival. Increased IL-21 has been found in the BM of patients with WM compared with healthy controls and IL-21 appears to be predominantly produced by T cells in the BM microenvironment. The receptor for IL-21 (IL-21R) is highly expressed on the surface of WM cells, suggesting that IL-21 may regulate the function of malignant WM cells. Further investigation revealed that IL-21 in the WM BM microenvironment stimulates cell proliferation and IgM secretion by malignant WM cells via an STAT-3–dependent pathway.[29] STAT5 was also found to be constitutively activated in WM and this activation is likely due to persistent cytokine signaling. Inhibition of STAT5 signaling was found to significantly decrease IgM production.[30]

BAFF is a TNF family member that is critical for maintenance of normal B-cell development and homeostasis, and BAFF has been found to be upregulated in the serum and BM of patients with WM.[31] BAFF is expressed by monocytes, macrophages, and dendritic cells, and potently induces B-cell proliferation and immunoglobulin secretion.[32] Malignant B cells in WM were found to bind soluble BAFF and variably express the receptors for B-cell activating factor (BAF), namely BAFF-R, TACI, and BCMA. BAFF, alone or in combination with cytokines, including IL-6, that induce immunoglobulin production, was found to increase IgM secretion by malignant B cells. Furthermore, BAFF was found to increase the viability and proliferation of malignant B cells from patients with WM.[31]

A further cytokine that has relevance in WM is macrophage inflammatory protein-1 alpha (MIP-1α). MIP-1α is increased in the serum of patients with WM and serum levels differ for different stages of the disease. MIP-1α is a member of CC chemokine family and is secreted by various cell types, including macrophages, lymphocytes, and dendritic cells. MIP-1α also activates osteoclast activity and is associated with bone disease in other plasma cell disorders. Although the presence of abnormal bone remodeling and increased bone resorption has been reported in WM, patients with WM do not typically have lytic bone disease, similar to that seen in multiple myeloma. In WM, the MIP-1α–induced osteoclast activity may be countered by an increase in osteoprotegerin, which has a role in bone formation. However, increases in MIP-1α in WM were found to correlate with disease activity, including increased serum β2-microglobulin and splenomegaly, implying that MIP-1α is relevant in the biology of WM.[33]

Finally, CXCL13 is a chemokine that is expressed in lymphoid organs by follicular dendritic cells and macrophages and is also produced by lymphoplasmacytic cells. Notably, CXCL13 attracts mast cells to the BM microenvironment. Recent data have suggested that CXCL13 levels vary in WM and appear lower among *CXCR4* frameshift but not *CXCR4* nonsense mutated patients versus those who were *CXCR4*^{WT}. An increased CXCL13 level was a strong predictor of achieving a response to BTK inhibition, and major responses to ibrutinib therapy were associated with deep suppression of CXCL13 levels.[34]

ANGIOGENESIS AND STROMAL ELEMENTS

Angiogenesis has been associated with disease progression and a poor prognosis in several hematological cancers.[35,36] Initial studies in symptomatic patients with WM reported that 30% of patients had increased microvascular density (MVD), whereas patients with IgM-monoclonal gammopathy of undetermined significance (IgM-MGUS) and patients with asymptomatic WM had reduced MVD in their BM. This suggested an angiogenic switch between asymptomatic and active phases of the disease.[37] Unfortunately, an increase in the MVD in the BM in WM correlated poorly with the extent of malignant cell infiltration and lacked a prognostic association with survival of patients with WM. Although angiogenesis appeared important once WM was present, it was unclear whether angiogenesis played a significant role in the progression of the disease.

However, increased angiogenesis in a group of patients with WM could be related to hypoxic conditions in the BM. Although hypoxia appears to prevent proliferation of

WM cells, it induces their dissemination and promotes homing in new BM niches.[38] Hypoxic WM cells lose their adhesion to the BMSCs and this effect is mediated by reduced E-cadherin expression on the surface of WM cells. In comparison with normoxic cells, hypoxic WM cells exhibit increased homing to the BM. This effect is mediated by increased expression of CXCL4 on WM cells, which promotes chemotaxis toward areas of increased SDF-1 expression, such as the BM.[28] This suggests that increased angiogenesis may overcome hypoxia in the BM and may thereby promote WM cell proliferation.

Changes in the expression level of angiogenic factors, including vascular endothelial growth factor (VEGF), VEGF-A, angiogenin, angiopoietin-1 (Ang-1), Ang-2, and basic fibroblast growth factor (bFGF), in patients with WM at different stages of their disease have been evaluated. Patients have been assessed before treatment onset, and then at the time of relapse or remission.[39] The data showed that serum levels of VEGF, VEGF-A, angiogenin, Ang-2, and bFGF are elevated, and Ang-1/Ang-2 ratio is reduced in all patients with WM irrespective of their phase of disease.[39] Serum angiogenin levels correlated with the active disease, and patients in remission had lower angiogenin levels when compared with untreated patients. Furthermore, Ang-1/Ang-2 ratios were inversely correlated with β2M and positively correlated with serum albumin levels.[39] These data indicate that angiogenic factors may be used as biomarkers to monitor disease progression. However, the mechanism by which each of these individual angiogenic factors contributes to disease progression in WM needs further investigation.

Furthermore, Eph-B2 may have a role in angiogenesis, as interactions between Eph-B2 on WM cells and EphrinB2 on the endothelial cells in the BM induces Ephrin-B2 phosphorylation. This subsequent phosphorylation of downstream signaling molecules in endothelial cells results in formation of new blood vessels.[21]

SUMMARY

Although our understanding of the role of BM microenvironment in WM has significantly increased in recent years, there are still many unknown factors that promote WM cell growth that need to be studied. Recent publications have provided insightful data on the BM constituents that support WM cells and explained in part which ligands or cell subpopulations promote malignant cell growth and proliferation, or stimulate immunoglobulin production (**Box 1**). WM cells have been shown to be in close contact

---

Box 1
Factors promoting the bone marrow niche in Waldenström macroglobulinemia

- Stromal derived factor-1 (SDF-1) induces increased migration of C-X-C chemokine receptor type 4 (CXCR4) expressing cells to the bone marrow

- Increased miR-155 modulates adhesion to fibronectin and promotes migration in response to SDF-1

- Increased hypoxia promotes colonization of the bone marrow niche

- Eph-B2/ephrin-B2 interaction enhances adhesion to endothelial and stromal cells

- Increased mast cells promote malignant cell growth through BAFF/APRIL/CD70/CD40 L signaling

- Cytokines, including CCL5, interleukin (IL)-6 and IL-21, promote malignant cell survival by means of a JAK/STAT/GLI2 signaling loop with BMSCs, mast cells, T cells, monocytes, macrophages, and endothelial cells. These cells directly stimulate malignant cell growth and promote IgM secretion by WM cells. Furthermore, cytokines and chemokines, including IL-6, IL-21, BAFF, and CCL5 also promote cell proliferation and induce IgM secretion. Future research will provide a more comprehensive understanding of the role of the BM microenvironment in WM and will allow for the design of effective therapeutic strategies that exploit the complex network of interactions in the environment on which WM cells rely.

REFERENCES

1. Monge J, Braggio E, Ansell SM. Genetic factors and pathogenesis of Waldenström's macroglobulinemia. Curr Oncol Rep 2013;15(5):450–6.

2. Treon SP, Xu L, Yang G, et al. MYD88 L265P somatic mutation in Waldenström's macroglobulinemia. N Engl J Med 2012;367(9):826–33.

3. Landgren O, Tageja N. MYD88 and beyond: novel opportunities for diagnosis, prognosis and treatment in Waldenström's macroglobulinemia. Leukemia 2014; 28(9):1799–803.

4. Lam LT, Wright G, Davis RE, et al. Cooperative signaling through the signal transducer and activator of transcription 3 and nuclear factor-{kappa}B pathways in subtypes of diffuse large B-cell lymphoma. Blood 2008;111(7):3701–13.

5. Krause DS, Scadden DT. A hostel for the hostile: the bone marrow niche in hematologic neoplasms. Haematologica 2015;100(11):1376–87.

6. Yang G, Zhou Y, Liu X, et al. A mutation in MYD88 (L265P) supports the survival of lymphoplasmacytic cells by activation of Bruton tyrosine kinase in Waldenström macroglobulinemia. Blood 2013;122(7):1222–32.

7. Hunter ZR, Xu L, Yang G, et al. The genomic landscape of Waldenström macroglobulinemia is characterized by highly recurring MYD88 and WHIM-like CXCR4 mutations, and small somatic deletions associated with B-cell lymphomagenesis. Blood 2014;123(11):1637–46.

8. Roccaro AM, Sacco A, Jimenez C, et al. C1013G/CXCR4 acts as a driver mutation of tumor progression and modulator of drug resistance in lymphoplasmacytic lymphoma. Blood 2014;123(26):4120–31.

9. Mendelson A, Frenette PS. Hematopoietic stem cell niche maintenance during homeostasis and regeneration. Nat Med 2014;20(8):833–46.

10. Smith JN, Calvi LM. Concise review: current concepts in bone marrow microenvironmental regulation of hematopoietic stem and progenitor cells. Stem Cells 2013;31(6):1044–50.

11. Tripodo C, Sangaletti S, Piccaluga PP, et al. The bone marrow stroma in hematological neoplasms–a guilty bystander. Nat Rev Clin Oncol 2011;8(8):456–66.

12. Sugiyama T, Nagasawa T. Bone marrow niches for hematopoietic stem cells and immune cells. Inflamm Allergy Drug Targets 2012;11(3):201–6.

13. Askmyr M, Quach J, Purton LE. Effects of the bone marrow microenvironment on hematopoietic malignancy. Bone 2011;48(1):115–20.

14. Ngo HT, Leleu X, Lee J, et al. SDF-1/CXCR4 and VLA-4 interaction regulates homing in Waldenström macroglobulinemia. Blood 2008;112(1):150–8.

15. Poulain S, Roumier C, Venet-Caillault A, et al. Genomic landscape of CXCR4 mutations in Waldenström macroglobulinemia. Clin Cancer Res 2016;22(6):1480–8.

16. Leleu X, Jia X, Runnels J, et al. The Akt pathway regulates survival and homing in Waldenström macroglobulinemia. Blood 2007;110(13):4417–26.

17. Roccaro AM, Sacco A, Chen C, et al. microRNA expression in the biology, prognosis, and therapy of Waldenström macroglobulinemia. Blood 2009;113(18): 4391–402.

18. Tournilhac O, Santos DD, Xu L, et al. Mast cells in Waldenström's macroglobulinemia support lymphoplasmacytic cell growth through CD154/CD40 signaling. Ann Oncol 2006;17(8):1275–82.

19. Ho AW, Hatjiharissi E, Ciccarelli BT, et al. CD27-CD70 interactions in the pathogenesis of Waldenström macroglobulinemia. Blood 2008;112(12):4683–9.

20. Jalali S, Price-Troska T, Villasboas JC, et al. Soluble PD-1 ligands regulate T-cell function in Waldenström's macroglobulinemia. Blood 2017;130:4034.

21. Azab F, Azab AK, Maiso P, et al. Eph-B2/ephrin-B2 interaction plays a major role in the adhesion and proliferation of Waldenström's macroglobulinemia. Clin Cancer Res 2012;18(1):91–104.

22. Konforte D, Simard N, Paige CJ. IL-21: an executor of B cell fate. J Immunol 2009; 182(4):1781–7.

23. Schneider P, MacKay F, Steiner V, et al. BAFF, a novel ligand of the tumor necrosis factor family, stimulates B cell growth. J Exp Med 1999;189(11):1747–56.

24. Akira S, Takeda K. Toll-like receptor signalling. Nat Rev Immunol 2004;4(7): 499–511.

25. Jefferies CA, Doyle S, Brunner C, et al. Bruton's tyrosine kinase is a Toll/interleukin-1 receptor domain-binding protein that participates in nuclear factor kappaB activation by Toll-like receptor 4. J Biol Chem 2003;278(28):26258–64.

26. Elsawa SF, Ansell SM. Cytokines in the microenvironment of Waldenström's macroglobulinemia. Clin Lymphoma Myeloma 2009;9(1):43–5.

27. Elsawa SF, Novak AJ, Ziesmer SC, et al. Comprehensive analysis of tumor microenvironment cytokines in Waldenström macroglobulinemia identifies CCL5 as a novel modulator of IL-6 activity. Blood 2011;118(20):5540–9.

28. Jackson DA, Smith TD, Amarsaikhan N, et al. Modulation of the IL-6 receptor alpha underlies GLI2-mediated regulation of Ig secretion in Waldenström macroglobulinemia cells. J Immunol 2015;195(6):2908–16.

29. Hodge LS, Ziesmer SC, Yang ZZ, et al. IL-21 in the bone marrow microenvironment contributes to IgM secretion and proliferation of malignant cells in Waldenström macroglobulinemia. Blood 2012;120(18):3774–82.

30. Hodge LS, Ziesmer SC, Yang ZZ, et al. Constitutive activation of STAT5A and STAT5B regulates IgM secretion in Waldenström's macroglobulinemia. Blood 2014;123(7):1055–8.

31. Elsawa SF, Novak AJ, Grote DM, et al. B-lymphocyte stimulator (BLyS) stimulates immunoglobulin production and malignant B-cell growth in Waldenström macroglobulinemia. Blood 2006;107(7):2882–8.

32. Moore PA, Belvedere O, Orr A, et al. BLyS: member of the tumor necrosis factor family and B lymphocyte stimulator. Science 1999;285(5425):260–3.

33. Terpos E, Anagnostopoulos A, Kastritis E, et al. Abnormal bone remodelling and increased levels of macrophage inflammatory protein-1 alpha (MIP-1alpha) in Waldenström macroglobulinaemia. Br J Haematol 2006;133(3):301–4.

34. Vos JM, Tsakmaklis N, Patterson CJ, et al. CXCL13 levels are elevated in patients with Waldenström macroglobulinemia, and are predictive of major response to ibrutinib. Haematologica 2017;102(11):e452–5.

35. Ribatti D, Scavelli C, Roccaro AM, et al. Hematopoietic cancer and angiogenesis. Stem Cells Dev 2004;13(5):484–95.

36. Ribatti D, Basile A, Ruggieri S, et al. Bone marrow vascular niche and the control of angiogenesis in multiple myeloma. Front Biosci 2014;19:304–11.

37. Rajkumar SV, Hayman S, Greipp PR. Angiogenesis in Waldenström's macroglobulinemia. Semin Oncol 2003;30(2):262–4.

38. Muz B, de la Puente P, Azab F, et al. Hypoxia promotes dissemination and colonization in new bone marrow niches in Waldenström macroglobulinemia. Mol Cancer Res 2015;13(2):263–72.

39. Anagnostopoulos A, Eleftherakis-Papaiakovou V, Kastritis E, et al. Serum concentrations of angiogenic cytokines in Waldenström macroglobulinaemia: the ratio of angiopoietin-1 to angiopoietin-2 and angiogenin correlate with disease severity. Br J Haematol 2007;137(6):560–8.

Familial Waldenström Macroglobulinemia
Families Informing Populations

Mary L. McMaster, MD[a,b],*

KEYWORDS

- Waldenström macroglobulinemia • Family studies • Cancer predisposition
- Environmental factors • Genetic susceptibility

KEY POINTS

- Family studies in Waldenström macroglobulinemia (WM) have provided the seminal observations leading to many aspects of the current understanding of WM susceptibility.
- The clinical phenotype of familial WM is broad; WM and lymphoplasmacytic lymphoma (LPL) coaggregate with other B-cell lymphoproliferative malignancies, immunoglobulin abnormalities, in vitro lymphocyte functional abnormalities, and autoimmune conditions.
- Immunoglobulin M (IgM) abnormalities are common within WM families and merit further evaluation, because they may eventually provide a basis for screening and prevention.
- A family history of WM/LPL has prognostic implications for WM patients.
- Family studies have provided evidence supporting not only genetic but also environmental factors contributing to WM predisposition; accumulating evidence supports the hypothesis that WM predisposition is complex and may reflect substantial genetic heterogeneity, an as-yet unrecognized common environmental exposure, and/or gene-environment interactions.

INTRODUCTION

Family studies are uniquely positioned to answer specific questions related to the cause and manifestations of Waldenström macroglobulinemia (WM) and have also frequently provided the initial observations that lead to definitive large-scale population studies with broadly applicable results. As such, family studies have occupied a

Disclosures: The author has no competing commercial or financial interests. Funding for the author's work described in this article is provided through the Intramural Research Program of the National Cancer Institute, National Institutes of Health, and U.S. Department of Health and Human Services.
^a Clinical Genetics Branch, Division of Cancer Epidemiology and Genetics, National Cancer Institute, National Institutes of Health, US Department of Health and Human Services, 9609 Medical Center Drive, Room 6E516, MSC 9772, Bethesda, MD 20892-9772, USA;
^b Commissioned Corps of the US Public Health Service, US Department of Health and Human Services, 330 C Street SW, Washington, DC 20416, USA
* 9609 Medical Center Drive, Room 6E516, MSC 9772, Bethesda, MD 20892-9772.
E-mail address: Mary.McMaster@nih.hhs.gov

Hematol Oncol Clin N Am 32 (2018) 787–809
https://doi.org/10.1016/j.hoc.2018.05.006
0889-8588/18/Published by Elsevier Inc.

pivotal role in WM research. The familial occurrence of WM in 2 brothers was first reported more than 50 years ago.[1] Familial clusters have subsequently been the subject of dedicated case reports[2–8] or embedded within larger family studies.[9–13] **Table 1** summarizes the most important studies of families published to date, some including extensive literature surveys.[14]

THE FAMILIAL WALDENSTRÖM MACROGLOBULINEMIA PHENOTYPE

Family studies first suggested that predisposition to WM encompasses a broader clinical phenotype than the occurrence of WM alone. The realization that the familial WM phenotype is complex was a critical observation, because characterizing the clinical phenotype may aid investigations of predisposition mechanisms by more precisely identifying at-risk individuals. Furthermore, from a clinical standpoint, familiality may have implications for screening, diagnosis, surveillance, and outcomes. Likewise, identification of modifiable environmental risk factors would be particularly useful for prevention strategies. Until better treatments and/or prevention strategies are developed for WM, identification of genetic factors mediating susceptibility may have limited practical clinical utility. Meanwhile, however, family studies also provide opportunities to study the natural history and pathophysiology of these disorders, which is also of value for nonfamilial cases.

Waldenström Macroglobulinemia Coaggregates with Related B-Cell Disorders

Family studies provided the initial suggestion that predisposition to WM includes susceptibility to related B-cell diseases, observing that WM sometimes clusters with other B-cell lymphoproliferative disorders (LPD), including chronic lymphocytic leukemia (CLL), other subtypes of non-Hodgkin lymphoma (NHL), and possibly multiple myeloma (MM), as well as with monoclonal gammopathy of undetermined significance (MGUS).[15–18] Ascertainment strategy and definitions critically influenced these studies' design and results.

Building on clues provided by families, population-based studies evaluated coaggregation of WM with other B-cell LPD. Because WM is a subset of lymphoplasmacytic lymphoma (LPL), population studies typically include both in order to increase power and to account for possible misclassification. These investigations confirmed that first-degree relatives of WM/LPL patients also have significantly increased risk of developing other B-cell malignancies, including CLL and NHL, but not HL or MM.[19,20] As illustrated in **Table 2**, the data supporting coaggregation are remarkably similar irrespective of the proband's diagnosis. Increased risk was also observed for MGUS, but immunoglobulin isotype data were unavailable. In contrast, other Scandinavian studies identified families containing both immunoglobulin G (IgG)/IgA and IgM disorders,[21,22] or increased risk of MM in certain inheritance patterns,[23] although the ascertainment scheme may have accounted for some of these results.

Conventional case-control studies have provided additional evidence supporting coaggregation of WM and other hematolymphoid diseases, including an international study that found a 64% increased risk for developing WM/LPL in individuals with a first-degree relative diagnosed with a hematologic malignancy.[24] Moreover, WM patients in a large single-center series reported a high prevalence (18.7%) of either WM or another B-cell disorder in first-degree relatives.[25] Taken together, WM definitely coaggregates with B-cell lymphoid disorders, whereas coaggregation of IgG/IgA and IgM disorders in the same family may occur. The relationship of MM to familial WM remains to be clarified. These data apply to predominantly white, northern European populations. Similar studies have not yet been conducted in other demographic groups.

Table 1
Reported familial clusters of Waldenström macroglobulinemia

| Year Reported and Reference | Fam | WM n | Other LPD n | Number of LPDs Occurring in Family | | Relationships Between All LPD Cases[a] | LPD Case Age and Gender[a] | Symptomatic WM |
| | | | | MGUS | | | | |
				IgM MGUS N	Non-IgM MGUS n			
Multiple-case WM families								
Massari et al,[1] 1962	1	2	0	1	0	Brothers–mother	61 M, 61 M, 83 F	Yes, yes
Coste et al,[10] 1964	1	2	0	0	0	Brother–sister	61 M, 54 F	Yes, nr
Gétaz and Staples,[2] 1977	1	2	0	0	0	Father–son	70 M, 47 M	Yes, yes
Youinou et al,[3] 1978	MIN	4	0	1	0	Brothers	61 M, 62 M, 64 M, 68 M	Nr
Blattner et al,[4] 1980	1	4	0	1[b]	0	Father–sons, daughter, grandson	77 M, 53 M, 42 M, 57 F, 52 M	No, yes, yes, no
Fine et al,[32] 1982	1	3	0	(2)[c]	0	Brother–brother, sister	61 M, (58)/65 M, (61)/ 76 F	Yes
Fine et al,[6] 1986	1	2	0	0	0	Monozygotic twins	75 M, 75 M	No, no
Renier et al,[7] 1989	1	4	0	0	0	Brothers[d]	76 M, 75 M, 72 M, 69 M	Yes, no, yes, yes
Renier et al,[7] 1989	1	2	0	0	0	Father–son	74 M, 47 M	Yes, yes
Renier et al,[7] 1989	1	2	0	0	0	Mother–daughter	74 F, 52 F	nr
Taleb et al,[8] 1991	1	2	0	0	0	Sisters	64 F, 43 F	Yes
Deshpande et al,[18] 1998	0047	2	1 MM; 1 HL[e]	0	1 IgG	Aunt–niece, granddaughter	72 F, 53 F, 49 F	nr
McMaster et al,[13] 2007	B	4	0	1	0	Mother–daughter, granddaughter, grandson, grandson	64 F, 51 F, 32 F, 57 M, 39 M	Yes, yes, yes, nr

(continued on next page)

Table 1
(continued)

				Number of LPDs Occurring in Family				
					MGUS			
Year Reported and Reference	Fam	WM n	Other LPD n	IgM MGUS N	Non-IgM MGUS n	Relationships Between All LPD Cases[a]	LPD Case Age and Gender[a]	Symptomatic WM
McMaster et al,[13] 2007	C	3	1 NHL[f]	2	0	Brother-sisters, brother, son	69 M, 69 F, nr F, 59 M, 34/ (52) M	Yes, yes, yes
Single-case WM + MGUS families								
Spengler et al,[59] 1966	IV	1	0	1	0	Father-daughter	69 M, 48 F	Yes
Seligmann et al,[12] 1967	ZA	1	0	1	0	Son-mother	56 M, 82 F	nr
Seligmann et al,[12] 1967	PE	1	0	1	0	Son-mother	41 M, 70 F	nr
Seligmann et al,[12] 1967	PO	1	0	1	0	Son-mother	57 M, 87 F	nr
Seligmann et al,[12] 1967	LA	1	0	1	0	Brother-brother	72 M, 70 M	nr
Seligmann et al,[12] 1967	MO	1	0	3	0	Sister-sister, son, daughter	65 F, 68 F, 54 M, 49 F	nr
Kalff and Hijmans,[34] 1969	Ru	1	0	1	0	Brother-sister	61 M, 71 F	Yes
Kalff and Hijmans,[34] 1969	Ho	1	0	1	0	Son-mother	53 M, 75 F	Yes
Renier et al,[7] 1989	1	1	0	1	2 NT	Mother-son	83 F, 42 M	nr
Linet et al,[60] 1993	A	1	0	1	0	Sister-sister	nr F, >76 F	nr
Zawadzki et al,[63] 1977	B	1	0	1	0	Father-daughter	nr M, >43 F	nr

Reference	Fam					Relationship	Sex/age at diagnosis	Male-to-male
Custodi et al,[29] 1995		1	1	0	0	**Brother**–sister	**73 M**, 70 F	nr
Manschot et al,[61] 2000		1	1	0	0	**Mother**–daughter	**70 F**, 50 F	Yes
Kalff and Hijmans,[34] 1969	Be	1	0	0	1 NT[g]	**Brother**–brother	**65 M**, 70 M	Yes
Kalff and Hijmans,[34] 1969	Ze	1	0	1	1 NT	**Brother**–brother–sister	**51 M**, 65 M, 57 F	No
Kalff and Hijmans,[34] 1969	Br	1	0	0	1 NT	**Uncle**–niece	**73 M**, 46 F	Yes
Kalff and Hijmans,[34] 1969	Wij	1	0	0	1 IgA	**Brother**–sister	**74 M**, 62 F	Yes
Kalff and Hijmans,[34] 1969	Vi	1	0	0	1 IgG	**2nd cousin**–2nd cousin	**75 M**, 85 F	Yes
Single-case WM + LPD families								
Kalff and Hijmans,[34] 1969	Hn	1	1 CLL; 1 NHL	1	1 IgG; 3 NT[g]	Complex, no male:male[h]	**80 M, 67 F, 62 M, 78 F**, 55 F, 49 M, 35 F, 55 F	nr
Fraumeni et al,[15] 1975		1	4 NHL; 1 HL; 1 ALL	0	0	Complex, no male:male[i]	**70 M, 75 M, 54 M, 50 M**, 68 F, 23 M, 5 M	Yes
Björnsson et al,[16] 1978		1	1 NHL; 1 MM[j]	2	0	**Sister**–brothers & niece	**71 F, 82 M, 77 M, 72 M**, 57 F	Yes
Steingrímsdóttir et al,[21] 2011		1	1 NHL; 3 MM	0	1 IgA; 1 NT	Complex, no male:male[k]	**F, F, M, M**, F, F (ages nr)	nr
Steingrímsdóttir et al,[21] 2011		3	2 NHL; 2 MM; 1 HL	0	2 IgG; 1 NT	Complex, no male:male[l]	**F, M, M, F, F**, M, M, F (ages nr)	nr

Abbreviations: ALL, acute lymphocytic leukemia; BMB, bone marrow biopsy; EP, electrophoresis; F, female; Fam, family; HL, Hodgkin lymphoma; LNB, lymph node biopsy; M, male; nr, not reported; NT, not typed.

[a] WM cases are shown in bold type. For subjects with MGUS and another LPD diagnosed at different ages, the age at MGUS diagnosis is shown in parentheses.

Complex relationships are also notated regarding whether male-to-male (male:male) inheritance was observed.

[b] Identified on follow-up of family (A) by McMaster and colleagues.[13]

[c] This family was originally reported as having 1 case of WM and 2 cases of IgM MGUS. The 2 patients with IgM MGUS progressed to WM 7 and 15 y later, respectively. Age at MGUS diagnosis is shown in parentheses.

[d] Bone marrow biopsy was reported only for the 72-year-old brother.

e The myeloma and Hodgkin lymphoma cases were both in the paternal bloodline of the IgG MGUS case, but not in the bloodline of either WM case. Their age and gender are not provided.

f A son of a WM case was diagnosed at age 34 with diffuse large B-cell lymphoma and was treated without recurrence during 21 y of follow-up. Eighteen years following his NHL diagnosis, he was discovered to have an IgM MGUS at age 52. Both diagnoses appear independently in the table.

g In Family Be, member II.2 (70-year-old man) is provisionally categorized as IgM MGUS based on having an IgM level 600% of the upper limit of the reference range, IgA level below the 95% tolerance limit for the reference range, normal IgG level, and a monoclonal protein that was not typed. In Family Hn, member IV.4 (35-year-old woman) is definitively categorized as IgM MGUS on the basis of a serum monoclonal protein typed as IgM, whereas member III.3 (55-year-old woman) is provisionally categorized as IgM MGUS based on an untyped monoclonal protein in the presence of an IgM level 230% of the upper limit of the reference range and normal IgA and IgG levels.

h In this 3-generation family, the WM case had a sister with IgG MGUS (or possibly myeloma), a granddaughter with IgM MGUS, and a brother and a daughter with untyped monoclonal proteins. The sister with IgG MGUS had a son with an untyped monoclonal protein.

i In this 4-generation family, the WM case had one sister and 3 brothers with NHL. The affected sister had a son with Hodgkin lymphoma and a great grandson with acute lymphocytic leukemia.

j MM developed in a niece and was reported by Ögmundsdóttir and colleagues.[17]

k In an extended family, the WM case had a sister with IgA MGUS and a father with untyped MGUS. On the maternal side were 2 cousins with NHL, 3 cousins with MM, and one cousin with acute myelogenous leukemia (AML).

l In an extended Icelandic pedigree, the WM case had a paternal aunt and cousin with MM, 2 paternal cousins with NHL, 3 paternal cousins with MGUS (IgG and untyped), one paternal cousin with HL, and one paternal cousin with AML.

Table 2
Relative risk for lymphoproliferative and plasma cell tumors among first-degree relatives of patients with Waldenström macroglobulinemia/lymphoplasmacytic lymphoma or other lymphoproliferative or plasma cell tumors or monoclonal gammopathy of undetermined significance, compared with relatives of matched controls

Proband Condition	WM/LPL OR (95% CI)	Non-Hodgkin Lymphoma OR (95% CI)	CLL OR (95% CI)	Hodgkin Lymphoma OR (95% CI)	MM OR (95% CI)	MGUS OR (95% CI)
WM/LPL	20[a] (4.1–98.4)	3.0 (2.0–4.4)	3.4 (1.7–6.6)	0.8 (0.3–2.2)	1.6 (0.8–3.2)	5.0 (1.3–18.9)
NHL	—	1.7 (1.4–2.2)	1.3 (0.9–1.9)	1.4 (1.0–2.0)	1.1 (0.8–1.5)	—
CLL	4.0 (2.0–8.2)	1.9 (1.5–2.3)	8.5 (6.1–11.7)	1.5 (0.96–2.3)	1.2 (0.9–1.8)	1.4 (0.9–2.2)
Hodgkin lymphoma	—	1.3 (0.9–1.8)	2.1 (1.2–3.8)	3.1 (1.8–5.3)	1.0 (0.6–1.8)	—
MM[b]	1.4 (0.7–2.8)	1.1 (0.9–1.4)	1.1 (0.8–1.7)	0.9 (0.6–1.4)	2.1 (1.6–2.9)	2.1 (1.5–3.1)
MGUS	2.0 (1.2–2.3)	1.1 (0.8–1.5)	2.0 (1.2–2.3)	1.3 (0.6–2.9)	2.9 (1.9–4.3)	2.8 (1.4–5.6)

Abbreviations: —, not applicable; CI, confidence interval; OR, odds ratio.

[a] Risk to relatives is highest for the proband's diagnosis, with the exception of MGUS, where relatives are at equally high risk for MM.

[b] A single study[23] subsequently reported a relationship between MM in a proband and risk of LPL/WM in the offspring. See text.

Adapted from Kristinsson SY, Goldin LR, Björkholm M, et al. Genetic and immune-related factors in the pathogenesis of lymphoproliferative and plasma cell malignancies. Haematologica 2009;94(11):1581–9; with permission.

Data are less compelling for coaggregation of WM and myeloid malignancies or solid tumors. For example, a clinically derived cohort of familial WM patients reported a proportional excess of myelopoietic cancers in their first- and second-degree relatives but conflicting data on solid tumors depending on the analytical methodology.[26,27] These observations were based on family report only and were not independently verified. In contrast, registry studies of WM/LPL patients found no increased risk for non-CLL leukemias in their relatives and conflicting results for solid tumors, conceivably because of multiple testing.[19,28] Thus, the preponderance of evidence supports an association of WM with other B-cell malignancies but not myeloid leukemias or solid tumors.

Autoimmunity and Familial Waldenström Macroglobulinemia

Family studies also initially indicated a relationship between WM and autoimmunity (**Table 3**), defined either clinically, ie, diagnosis of a symptomatic autoimmune disorder, or subclinically, through demonstration of high titers of autoantibodies without associated symptoms. Although reporting instances of clinical autoimmune disease (eg, rheumatoid arthritis) in family members, early family studies focused primarily on subclinical manifestations. A variety of autoantibodies were evaluated in a subset of multiple-case families and in families of sporadic WM. Frequency of autoantibodies in relatives of WM cases ranges from 4% to 25%.[3,4,6,11,15,17,29] A clinical diagnosis of autoimmune disease was rarely reported in early studies, although in only one study were relevant medical history data explicitly sought and validated.[4] More recently, investigators have reported validated autoimmune disease in relatives among 5 of 12 (42%) WM families.[22] Unfortunately, the lack of controls in most studies precluded definite conclusions. Moreover, the prevalence of many autoantibodies in the general population is unknown, although some (eg, antithyroid antibodies and low-level rheumatoid factor) are known to be relatively common among apparently healthy subjects.

Nonetheless, these family-based observations provided the impetus for a large population-based study to evaluate familial predisposition to diagnosed autoimmune disease and WM/LPL. In this registry-based case-control study, family history of specific autoimmune diseases was significantly associated with risk of WM/LPL.[30] It did not include a laboratory screening arm to assess subclinical manifestations of autoimmunity.

Overall, these findings suggest that an underlying immunoregulatory defect is present in WM families. Because immune dysfunction is a known predisposing factor for lymphoma, carefully designed studies will be required to determine whether the immune dysfunction itself predisposes to WM or a more general immunogenetic defect exists that may manifest as malignancy, autoimmunity, or both.

Immunoglobulin M Monoclonal Gammopathy of Undetermined Significance in Waldenström Macroglobulinemia Families

One of the most interesting discoveries to arise from detailed evaluation of WM families is the frequent occurrence of other immunoglobulin abnormalities in apparently unaffected relatives of WM patients. The most striking of these is IgM MGUS (**Table 4**). The very first description of a WM family noted asymptomatic IgM monoclonal gammopathy in the healthy parent of 2 WM patients.[1] Subsequent family studies revealed IgM MGUS as a frequent finding in WM families,[3,4,12,22] although its prevalence remains undefined. IgM MGUS has been recognized independently as a risk factor for subsequent development of WM and other B-cell LPD, progressing to malignancy at a rate of 1.5% per year.[31] In the initial family report, monoclonal gammopathy was transient. However, long-term follow-up studies have shown that relatives with IgM MGUS may be at high

Table 3
Autoimmunity associated with familial Waldenström macroglobulinemia

Year Reported & Reference	Families Studied (n)	WM Cases (n)	Unaffected Relatives Studied 1st Degree/Total (n)	Age Range	Findings Related to Autoimmunity in Relatives Clinical n	Disease (n)	Lab n	Laboratory Assays Reported	Abnormal Assays (n)
Studies of Aggregated WM Families									
Seligmann et al,[11] 1966; Seligmann et al,[12] 1967[a]	63	65	192/216	5–87	—	—	46	AyG, AGA, ANA, ATA, CA	AyG
Linet et al,[60] 1993[b]	8	8	45/45	>9[c]	5	nr	—	—	—
Studies of Individual WM Families									
Fraumeni et al,[15] 1975	1	1	2/9	42–64	3	Raynaud (1), possible RA (2)	—	—	—
Youinou et al,[3] 1978	1	4	8/35	1–65	0	n.a.	5	ADA, RF AMC, AMt, ANA, APA,	ADA (1); RF (4) RF (3); ATG (2); ATM(3); AMC (2)
Blattner et al,[4] 1980	1	4	13/16	nr	2	Hashimoto thyroiditis (2)	8	ASM, ATG, ATM, RF AMt, ANA, APA, ARA,	—
Renier et al,[7] 1989	1	4	2/12	20–63	—	—	2	ASM, ATG, ATM, RF	ANA (1); ATG (1)
Renier et al,[7] 1989	1	2	nr/2	nr	0	n.a.	0	nr	nr

(continued on next page)

Table 3
(continued)

Year Reported & Reference	Families Studied n	WM Cases n	Unaffected Relatives Studied		Findings Related to Autoimmunity in Relatives				
			1st Degree/Total n	Age Range	Clinical		Lab	Laboratory Assays	Abnormal Assays (n)
					n	Disease (n)	n	Reported	
Ögmundsdóttir et al,[17] 1994	1	1	1/34	nr	—	—	1	ANA, RF	ANA (1)
Custodi et al,[29] 1995	1	1	4/4	25–70	—	—	1	ATG, RF, cryo	ATG (1)
Brandefors et al,[22] 2016	12	19	45/59	nr	5	RA (2); Sjögren syndrome (1); hypothyroidism (1); PMR (1)	—	—	—

Abbreviations: —, evaluation or assay not performed; ADA, anti-DNA antibodies; AGA, antigastric antibodies; A-IF, anti-intrinsic factor; AMC, antimyocardial antibodies; AMt, antimitochondrial antibodies; ANA, antinuclear antibodies; ANP, antinucleoprotein antibodies; APA, antiparietal cell antibodies; ARA, antireticulin antibodies; ASM, antismooth muscle antibodies; ATA, antithyroid antibodies; ATG, antithyroglobulin; ATM, antithyroid microsomal; AγG, anti-γ-globulin factors; CA, cold agglutinin titers; cryo, cryoglobulins; Lab, laboratory assays; n.a., not applicable; nr, not reported; PMR, polymyalgia rheumatica; RA, rheumatoid arthritis; RF, rheumatoid factor.

ª Includes 2 multiple-case WM families reported by Massari and colleagues[1] and Coste and colleagues,[10] respectively, and one WM + MGUS family reported by Vannotti.[9] Although 216 relatives were studied, immunoglobulin levels were reported only for the 192 first-degree relatives.

ᵇ The study was based on the families of 31 WM patients. Results were reported as OR for the aggregate study. Individual results were reported for 45 relatives (all first-degree) from 8 families and are included here.

ᶜ Year of birth was reported. For this table, age was estimated using date of birth and last date of study entry (December 31, 1983).

Table 4
Immunoglobulin abnormalities associated with familial Waldenström macroglobulinemia

					Number of Relatives Found to Have Immunoglobulin Abnormalities																
					Monoclonal Component				Polyclonal Ig Increase						Decrease Ig						
			Relatives										Multiple Ig						Multiple Ig		
Year Reported & Reference	Families Studied n	WM Cases n	1st degree/Total n	Age Range	Any n	IgM n	Non-IgM n	Type	Any n	IgM n	IgA n	IgG n	Incl IgM n	Excl IgM n	Any n	IgM n	IgA n	IgG n	Incl IgM n	Excl IgM n	Ig Abnormalities, Other or NOS n
Studies of Aggregated WM Families																					
Seligmann,[11] 1966; Seligmann et al,[12] 1967	63	65	192/216	5–87	6	6	0	—	34	10	17	0	5	2	42	18	15	0	7	2	3
Kalff & Hijmans,[34] 1969[a]	12	12	72/282	>10	11	3	8	1 IgA; 2 IgG; 5 NT	46	37	11	9	5	2	14	2	6	0	4	3	1 (↑M↑G↓A)
Line et al,[60] 1993	31	31	>45/109	>9[b]	2	2	0	—	18	2	7	5	0	4	6	0	5	0	0	1	0
McMaster et al,[13] 2007[c]	3	10	25/25	16–80	5	5	0	—	9	5	0	0	0	4	2	0	0	0	2	0	0
Brandefors et al,[22] 2016	12	19	45/59	nr	12[d]	8	4	3 IgG; 1 FLC	4	2	2	0	0	0	6	1	1	4	0	0	nr
Studies of Individual WM Families																					
Fine et al,[5] 1966	1	1	7/27	1–67	2	2	0	—	13	13	0	0	0	0	0	0	0	0	0	0	0
Spengler et al,[59] 1966	1	1	4/4	nr	1	1	0	—	0	0	—	—	—	0	0	0	—	—	—	—	—

(continued on next page)

Table 4 (continued)

Year Reported & Reference	Families Studied n	WM Cases n	Relatives 1st degree/Total n	Age Range	Monoclonal Component Any n	IgM n	Non-IgM n	Non-IgM Type	Polyclonal Ig Increase Any n	IgM n	IgA n	IgG n	Multiple Ig Incl IgM n	Multiple Ig Excl IgM n	Decrease Ig Any n	IgM n	IgA n	IgG n	Multiple Ig Incl IgM n	Multiple Ig Excl IgM n	Ig Abnormalities, Other or NOS n
Williams et al,[62] 1967	1	1	nr/6	nr	0	0	0	—	—	—	—	—	—	—	—	—	—	—	—	—	—
Fraumeni et al,[15] 1975	1	1	2/9	42–64	0	0	0	—	3	3	0	0	0	0	0	0	0	0	0	0	0
Zawadzki et al,[63] 1977	1	1	5/5	30–98	2	2	0	—	—	—	—	—	—	—	—	—	—	—	—	—	—
Youinou et al,[3] 1978	1	4	8/35	1–65	1	1	0	—	3	3	0	0	0	13	0	2	11	0	0	0	0
Björnsson et al,[16] 1978	1	1	5/49	nr	2	2	0	—	12	9	1	0	0	2	0	0	0	0	0	0	0
Fine et al,[6] 1986[e]	1	2	6/6	nr	0	0	0	—	0	0	—	0	—	0	0	0	—	0	—	0	0
Renier et al,[7] 1989	1	4	2/12	20–63	0	0	0	—	6	1	1	2	1	1	0	0	0	0	0	0	0
Renier et al,[7] 1989	1	1	2/4	nr	1	1	0	—	0	0	0	0	0	0	0	0	0	0	0	0	0

Number of Relatives Found to Have Immunoglobulin Abnormalities

Renier et al,[7] 1989	1	2	nr/2	nr	nr	0	0	0	—	0	0	0	0	0	0	0	0	0	0	0
Renier et al,[7] 1989	1	1	nr/4	nr	nr	0	3	1	2	2 NT	0	0	0	0	0	0	0	0	0	0
Taleb et al,[8] 1991	1	2	7/7	8–67	8-67	0	0	0	0	—	4	4	0	0	0	0	0	0	0	0
Custodi et al,[29] 1995	1	1	4/4	25–70	25-70	1	1	0	0	—	0	0	0	1	0	1	0	0	0	2(↑IgE)

Abbreviations: —, assay not performed; abnl, abnormality; excl, excluding; FLC, free light chain; Ig, immunoglobulin(s); incl, including; NOS, not otherwise specified; nr, not reported; NT, not typed.

a The study included 353 relatives of 23 patients with IgM monoclonal gammopathy. Patients were categorized as having definite WM (n = 11), possible WM (n = 6), IgM monoclonal gammopathy associated with other cancers (n = 4) or autoimmune disease (n = 1) and "benign essential monoclonal gammopathy" (n = 1). Results were reported for 282 relatives from 12 families having WM, including 6 definite WM and 6 possible WM. Results are also presented for families with MGUS and autoimmune-related IgM monoclonal gammopathy.

b Year of birth was reported only for families with identified abnormalities. For this table, age was estimated using date of birth and last date of study entry (December 31, 1983).

c Includes the family reported by Blattner and colleagues.[4]

d IgM MGUS was included in the definition of familial WM in this study; 2 families had only 1 case of WM and one or more cases of IgM MGUS, which may bias the results.

e Subjects were tested for IgG levels only.

risk for progression to WM, perhaps at a rate exceeding that of progression of IgM MGUS to WM in the general population. The first such family contained 2 relatives with IgM monoclonal gammopathy who progressed to WM in 7 and 15 years, respectively.[32] A later study of 3 multiple-case US WM families with a median follow-up of 17 years documented IgM monoclonal gammopathy in 24% of relatives, with 3 subsequently diagnosed with WM, 3 with progressive increases in their monoclonal IgM, and one with persistent, stable IgM monoclonal gammopathy.[13] In an Icelandic family, progression to WM was observed in 2 cases with IgM MGUS at 3 and 6 years, respectively.[17,21] Four of the 5 families in these reports were unusual in having many members affected with WM, so it is unclear whether the observed risk of progression applies to all WM families. These observations together have established IgM MGUS as a precursor condition within the familial WM spectrum. Active areas of research include establishing the prevalence of IgM monoclonal gammopathy in WM families, defining the spectrum of outcomes, estimating the risk of progression, and developing screening guidelines for families. In addition, the consequences of qualitative or small-volume IgM monoclonal gammopathy (defined as the presence of a monoclonal band on immunofixation that is not accompanied by a measurable M-spike on protein electrophoresis) have yet to be defined.[33]

Other Immunoglobulin Abnormalities in Waldenström Macroglobulinemia Families

Relatives of WM patients may have other immunoglobulin abnormalities in addition to IgM monoclonal gammopathy (see **Table 4**). Several studies of multiple-case WM or WM/LPD families or presumed nonfamilial WM have confirmed abnormalities affecting all major immunoglobulin classes, IgM, IgA, and IgG.[3,7,8,12,13,15–17,22,34]

These observations suggest predisposition to WM may actually reflect a more generalized predisposition to immune dysregulation. Because the overall prevalence of subclinical immunoglobulin abnormalities in the general population is unknown, it is difficult to conclude that they are more frequent in the familial context. For example, polyclonal immunoglobulin elevations were more frequent in first-degree relatives of WM cases compared with non–bloodline controls (ie, spouses), although the difference was not significant.[13] In contrast, there was no difference in the prevalence of immunoglobulin deficiencies in relatives versus controls in these families. Higher prevalence of polyclonal immunoglobulin elevations might reflect an underlying condition of polyclonal B-cell activation, which would accord with the findings reported by Steingrimsdóttir and colleagues.[21] All these studies have been limited by potential confounding; it is known, for example, that immunoglobulin concentrations are influenced by age, race, and gender.[35,36] Furthermore, relatives typically have not been medically evaluated for possible known immunodeficiency syndromes or followed longitudinally to confirm that the immunoglobulin abnormalities are persistent over time or to document outcomes.

The Hyperresponder Phenotype

Blood levels of immunoglobulins and autoantibodies reflect B-cell function and activity in vivo. The first report of in vitro studies on lymphocytes from members of WM families showed impaired responses to stimulation with phytohemagglutinin, a T-cell mitogen.[15] Extensive in vitro testing of peripheral blood lymphocytes from unaffected relatives in Icelandic families led to the identification of the hyperresponder phenotype. The hyperresponder phenotype is defined as increased production of immunoglobulins, IgG and IgM, in pokeweed–mitogen-stimulated cultures. Seventeen hyperresponders were identified in 4 families, 12 of them in one large family where

40 persons were tested.[17,21] Lymphocytes from hyperresponders show enhanced survival in stimulated cultures, and this is associated with increased levels of the anti-apoptotic protein Bcl-2.[37]

PRESENTATION AND OUTCOMES OF FAMILIAL WALDENSTRÖM MACROGLOBULINEMIA

Historical survey of 40 years of accumulated individual family reports suggested that most features of the WM disease process in familial WM did not differ substantially from that expected based on review of the literature.[14] Exceptions included observations that familial WM patients were diagnosed nearly a decade younger than sporadic cases and were much more likely to be men.[38] However, other disease characteristics, including presenting symptoms and signs, and laboratory features accorded with expectations for nonfamilial WM. In vitro studies revealed no distinguishing features of the IgM molecules isolated from familial patients. Limited cytogenetic analyses found no chromosomal abnormalities that discriminated familial from nonfamilial cases.[3,8,11,39,40]

More recent studies have focused on cohorts of patients who report a family history of WM or other B-cell LPD and have included as controls nonfamilial WM cases and sometimes unaffected relatives.[25,41] Notable findings were that familial patients were more likely than nonfamilial to present with a high IgM level (>3000 mg/dL) and a nonsignificant increase in tumor burden at referral. Otherwise, there was no difference in age at diagnosis, gender, onset, or spectrum of symptoms, prior history of MGUS, extent of bone marrow involvement at diagnosis, lymphadenopathy, splenomegaly, concomitant IgA and IgG hypogammaglobulinemia, anemia, thrombocytopenia or beta-2-microglobulin. Cytogenetic analysis, including more sensitive fluorescence in situ hybridization (FISH) studies of a subset of patients, also confirmed no significant differences between groups. In addition, time from diagnosis to first treatment did not differ between groups, with insufficient events to permit meaningful survival analysis.

Thus, the question of age at onset remains unresolved, and no clinical features appear to reliably differentiate familial from nonfamilial WM at disease presentation. Initially, familial WM was thought to be associated with a more indolent course, at least in its early stages, based on the observation that higher IgM levels at referral were not accompanied by more severe symptoms, signs, or other laboratory abnormalities. Newer data in hospital and population studies, however, refute this and instead show that family history is associated with poorer outcomes, with familial patients having shorter time to progression and time to next therapy than nonfamilial patients, with too few events to assess survival.[42] Although the subset analysis was limited by small numbers and relatively shorter follow-up, this observation may have important clinical implications and deserves additional study. Similarly, in a recent population-based analysis of the impact of familial disease on survival,[43] overall survival in WM/LPL patients having a first-degree relative with any lymphoproliferative disease was significantly inferior to patients without a family history. This finding could not be explained by differences in age or calendar period of diagnosis between groups; however, detailed clinical data (eg, bone marrow results or treatment) were not available. Based on these findings, family history information should be routinely collected from all patients on clinical trials so that confirmatory analyses can be performed.

PREDISPOSITION TO WALDENSTRÖM MACROGLOBULINEMIA
Environmental Factors in Familial Waldenström Macroglobulinemia

Interestingly, family studies were among the first to investigate the role of environment in WM predisposition. Early family studies focused on the possible role of a disordered immune response to a shared antigen exposure within a family. Some of these studies applied extensive investigation of the characteristics of the IgM molecule in familial WM and IgM MGUS patients.[3,6,7,11] In families where IgM was characterized, light chain typing was discordant among the cases,[7,11] including affected monozygotic twins,[6] and related patients differed in other molecular characteristics of IgM, including light chain mobility, immunoglobulin allotyping, or idiotypic determinants,[3,11] suggesting that familial cases could not be explained by clonal B-cell expansion in response to some common exposure. Subsequently, familial cases were found to be more likely than nonfamilial cases to report a history of certain environmental exposures, including farming, organic solvents, and wood dust.[41] Risk of WM was later associated with a variety of environmental exposures in a case-control study.[24] Thus, the findings overall suggest that predisposition to WM is complex and may reflect an interaction of host and environmental factors.

Genetic Factors in Predisposition to Waldenström Macroglobulinemia

Confirmation of WM familial clustering at the population level provided the foundation for studies directed at unraveling the genetic basis for WM. These efforts have proved challenging. Initially, the most commonly observed pedigree configuration consisted of 2 affected siblings, consistent with autosomal recessive inheritance. As the National Cancer Institute WM family registry accumulated increasing numbers of families, multiple pedigree configurations were observed (**Fig. 1**). The occurrence of cases in multiple generations strengthens the argument for inherited factors rather than shared environment. Another potential explanation for single-generation clusters is that affected individuals in earlier generations may have been undiagnosed or misclassified. The diversity of reported inheritance patterns involving cases in one or more generations suggests that several different genes might be involved, and the coaggregation of different B-cell disorders implies that causative genes may be operating at the level of lymphopoietic stem cells. In any case, early evidence indicates that any susceptibility gene or genes may have low penetrance and possibly pleiotropic effects.

Cytogenetics

Early cytogenetic studies in family clusters were inconclusive.[3,8,39] Investigators prospectively using multiple methodologies to systematically examine bone marrow and peripheral blood from familial WM and IgM MGUS patients found a small number of recurrent deletion events.[40] However, only one abnormality was found in both tumor and peripheral blood mononuclear cells, and none were seen in bone marrow cells from IgM MGUS patients or were shared between WM patients from the same family. Another prospective study of bone marrow cytogenetics in familial WM patients found del6q21 by FISH in tumor cells in a high proportion of both familial and nonfamilial patients but did not assess the germline.[25] Thus, to date, cytogenetic studies have not identified any regions that may contain WM predisposition genes.

Linkage and Candidate Gene Association Studies

Genome-wide linkage analysis is an established tool for identifying chromosomal regions that may harbor susceptibility genes that cosegregate with disease in informative families. Genome-wide linkage was conducted in 11 well-characterized, informative high-risk WM families using densely spaced microsatellite markers to localize susceptibility genes with parallel analyses either including or excluding IgM MGUS as a phenotype indicating affected status.[44] The 2 key findings included: (1) evidence for linkage to 4 chromosomal regions argued strongly for potential genetic

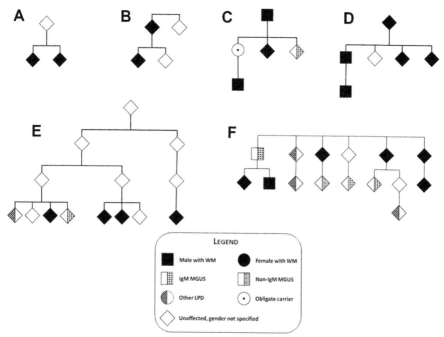

Fig. 1. The diversity of WM pedigrees. (*A*) One of the most common configurations: a family containing 2 affected individuals, in this case parent and offspring. All possible gender configurations, that is, father to son or daughter, and mother to son or daughter, have been observed. (*B*) Another common configuration consisting of affected siblings. (*C*) An autosomal dominant pattern of inheritance, with 3 generations of male-to-male transmission. (*D*) A family that demonstrates incomplete penetrance. (*E*) A pedigree configuration compatible with autosomal recessive transmission. (*F*) This pedigree demonstrates that a variety of LPDs may be found in different combinations in some families. Families C, E, and F are remarkable for the large number of individuals affected with WM. However, there is often insufficient information about older generations to determine whether earlier family members may have been affected.

heterogeneity; (2) IgM MGUS was clearly shown for the first time to be part of the familial WM spectrum, because including it strengthened evidence for linkage.

Liang and colleagues[45] used a candidate gene approach to genotype single nucleotide polymorphisms (SNPs) in genes implicated in apoptosis/cell-cycle regulation, DNA repair, immune response, T-helper cell type 1/2 subsets, tumor necrosis factor/nuclear factor kappa B pathways, and oxidative stress based on data from genome-wide association studies (GWAS) of NHL. Twenty SNPs in 5 genes (*BCL6, IL10, IL6, IL8Ra,* and *TNFSF10*) were significantly associated with WM following correction for multiple comparisons, again suggesting that WM is characterized by genetic heterogeneity.

Other Genetic Markers of Waldenström Macroglobulinemia Predisposition

HLA typing has been undertaken in a small number of families. HLA A9 was expressed in 2 families,[3,4] but no haplotype was shared among families. The *A9-B8-DRw3* haplotype cosegregated with both WM and autoimmune thyroid disease in one family.[4] This observation is interesting in retrospect, because this haplotype has since been more extensively characterized and identified as the HLA 8.1 ancestral haplotype (AH), which is carried by 10% of Northern Europeans and also includes the *TNF* locus.[46] The AH 8.1 is associated with many autoimmune diseases, including some that are also risk factors for WM,[24] and has been shown to interact with a variety of NHL risk factors, including family history, to modulate NHL risk.[47] In addition, the *TNF* G308A variant allele has been associated with diffuse large B-cell lymphoma and marginal zone lymphoma.[48] Systematic evaluation of more WM families will determine whether the cooccurrence of the AH 8.1 with WM and autoimmune disease is a true and recurrent association.

Some investigators have focused on the targets of paraproteins as risk factors for development of IgM MGUS and WM. Paraproteins from 11% of patients with either IgM MGUS or WM reacted specifically with hyperphosphorylated paratarg-y (pP-7).[49] Constitutive hyperphosphorylation of these proteins may be inherited as an autosomal dominant trait in some families, suggesting that chronic antigenic stimulation by lifelong exposure to an inherited aberrant autoantigen could account for familial clustering of WM. Cosegregation of WM and pP-7 carrier state has not yet been demonstrated as a systematic recurrent event in multiple-case WM families.

Research on the role of stroma and extracellular matrix in MM led to the discovery of the gene coding for hyaluron synthase 1, *HAS1*, as a potentially important gene in B-cell–derived malignancies, showing associations with both somatic and germ-line mutations.[50,51] The effects are not related to the role of *HAS1* in synthesis of extracellular matrix but instead relate to identified genetic variants in introns that lead to alternative splicing yielding proteins with intracellular effects. Transfection with these *HAS1* variants induces a malignant phenotype, and the variants show different intracellular distribution and interaction with the cytoskeleton.[52] SNPs in *HAS1* intron 3, associated with B-cell–derived malignancies, had significantly increased frequency in members of single family affected with WM, MM, MGUS, or the hyperresponder phenotype.[53]

Massively Parallel Genomic Technologies

Massively parallel sequencing tools comprise a strategy to discover whether rare, high-penetrance germline mutations contribute to WM susceptibility. Whole-genome sequencing of tumor tissue led to the discovery of *MYD88* mutation as a key somatic event in WM tumorigenesis.[54] Targeted sequencing showed the *MYD88* L265P mutation is not present in the germline of familial WM patients, effectively eliminating it as a WM susceptibility gene.[55] Identification of potentially deleterious rare variants in 2 genes cosegregating in affected members of a single family and apparently enriched in familial versus nonfamilial WM cases demonstrates the power and challenges of this approach.[56] Such mutations have been convincingly demonstrated in Mendelian disorders. However, whether recurrent high-penetrance disease-related mutations can be identified in complex diseases such as WM, even within large, multigenerational families, remains to be seen. Preliminary data suggest there are significant challenges in the conduct and interpretation of large sequencing studies in cancer-prone families generally[57] and that genetic heterogeneity may be extensive in WM/LPL.[58] Genomic sequencing will be best used by incorporating it into multidisciplinary studies using multiple technological approaches, such as epigenetic and expression studies and RNA sequencing in addition to the strategies already discussed here.

The evidence for genetic heterogeneity suggests a likely role for more common genetic variation in WM cause. However, as yet no GWAS assessing the role of common genetic polymorphisms in WM susceptibility has been performed, likely because of the difficulty in assembling an adequately powered sample of WM cases for study.

Once such a sample is accumulated, it will be interesting to discover whether GWAS findings resemble those in other B-cell malignancies. Results from GWAS may also address known biologically plausible candidate genes, potential differences between familial and sporadic WM cases, and other relevant subgroup issues.

SUMMARY

Family studies have been pivotal in the following:

- Providing opportunities for long-term observation of the natural history of disease progression, identifying additional risk factors, refining the clinical phenotype, and guiding gene-discovery and other efforts aimed at unraveling the molecular determinants of WM
- Providing the initial observations and impetus for generalizable population-based studies regarding many aspects of WM, including familial clustering of WM/LPL and coaggregation of WM with other B-cell and autoimmune disorders
- Recognizing IgM-MGUS as a precursor condition for WM and may ultimately provide insights into determinants of disease progression

Furthermore, in the research context, screening of high-risk family members for IgM MGUS could identify a cohort that may benefit from future prevention strategies. Additional work in WM families may therefore hold the key to answering 2 important questions: (1) identifying the link between age-related changes in the immune system and monoclonal gammopathies, and (2) understanding what determines risk of malignant progression, thereby paving the way toward prevention studies.

Notably, family studies also provided some of the preliminary evidence for a role for environmental exposures in WM development. The precise contributions of environmental and genetic factors to WM predisposition remain undefined. Much of the available evidence, including familial clustering, population data, associated findings in relatives of patients with WM, and some genetic data, supports the hypothesis that genetic factors are important determinants in the development of WM. Whether such factors are directly responsible for WM or operate through intermediary conditions such as immunodeficiency is less clear. In WM, the acquired L265P activating mutation in the *MYD88* gene, found in a very high proportion of patients regardless of family history, is clearly a major determining event providing selective advantage. However, no data support the L265P mutation as a likely germline mutation candidate in families predisposed to developing IgM MGUS and WM. Meanwhile, mutations in other rare, high-penetrance genes and polymorphisms affecting more common, low-penetrance genes may be identified and will require careful study to delineate their contribution to WM susceptibility. Both clinical and genetic studies suggest that there may be extensive genetic heterogeneity in this disease, and a role for environmental factors operating through chronic antigenic stimulation remains viable. Systematic family studies can continue to inform the understanding of whether WM susceptibility may be mediated by highly penetrant rare gene variants, common variants in multiple genes, variants in regulatory regions, or through gene-environment interactions.

REFERENCES

1. Massari R, Fine JM, Metais R. Waldenström's macroglobulinæmia observed in two brothers. Nature 1962;196:176–8.
2. Gétaz EP, Staples WG. Familial Waldenström's macroglobulinaemia: a case report. S Afr Med J 1977;51:891–2.

3. Youinou P, Le Goff P, Saleun JP, et al. Familial occurrence of monoclonal gamma-pathies. Biomedicine 1978;28(4):226–32.
4. Blattner WA, Garber JE, Mann DL, et al. Waldenström's macroglobulinemia and autoimmune disease in a family. Ann Intern Med 1980;93:830–2.
5. Fine JM, Massari R, Boffa GA, et al. Macroglobulinémie à caractère familial présente chez trois sujets d'une même fratrie. Transfusion (Paris) 1966;9(4):333–41.
6. Fine JM, Muller JY, Rochu D, et al. Waldenström's macroglobulinemia in monozygotic twins. Acta Med Scand 1986;220(4):369–73.
7. Renier G, Ifrah N, Chevailler A, et al. Four brothers with Waldenstrom's macroglobulinemia. Cancer 1989;64(7):1554–9.
8. Taleb N, Tohme A, Abi JD, et al. Familial macroglobulinemia in a Lebanese family with two sisters presenting Waldenström's disease. Acta Oncol 1991;30(6):703–5.
9. Vannotti A. Etude clinique dun cas de macroglobulinemia de Waldenstrom a caractere familial, associe a des trouble endocriniens. Schweiz Med Wochenschr 1963;93:1744–6.
10. Coste F, Massais P, Menkes C. Un cas de macroglobulinemia. Rev Rhum Mal Osteoartic 1964;31:37–9.
11. Seligmann M. A genetic predisposition to Waldenstrom's macroglobulinaemia. Acta Med Scand 1966;179(S445):140–6.
12. Seligmann M, Danon F, Mihaesco C, et al. Immunoglobulin abnormalities in families of patients with Waldenström's macroglobulinemia. Am J Med 1967;43(1):66–83.
13. McMaster ML, Csako G, Giambarresi TR, et al. Long-term evaluation of three multiple-case Waldenström macroglobulinemia families. Clin Cancer Res 2007; 13(17):5063–9.
14. McMaster ML. Familial Waldenstrom's macroglobulinemia. Semin Oncol 2003; 30(2):146–52.
15. Fraumeni JF, Wertelecki W, Blattner WA, et al. Varied manifestations of a familial lymphoproliferative disorder. Am J Med 1975;59(1):145–51.
16. Björnsson OG, Arnason A, Gudmunosson S, et al. Macroglobulinaemia in an Icelandic family. Acta Med Scand 1978;203(4):283–8.
17. Ögmundsdóttir HM, Jóhannesson GM, Sveinsdóttir S, et al. Familial macroglobulinaemia: hyperactive B-cells but normal natural killer function. Scand J Immunol 1994;40(2):195–200.
18. Deshpande HA, Hu XP, Marino P, et al. Anticipation in familial plasma cell dyscrasias. Br J Haematol 1998;103(3):696–703.
19. Altieri A, Bermejo JL, Hemminki K. Familial aggregation of lymphoplasmacytic lymphoma with non-Hodgkin lymphoma and other neoplasms. Leukemia 2005; 19(12):2342–3.
20. Kristinsson SY, Björkholm M, Goldin LR, et al. Risk of lymphoproliferative disorders among first-degree relatives of lymphoplasmacytic lymphoma/Waldenstrom macroglobulinemia patients: a population-based study in Sweden. Blood 2008; 112(8):3052–6.
21. Steingrimsdóttir H, Einarsdóttir HK, Haraldsdóttir V, et al. Familial monoclonal gammopathy: hyper-responsive B cells in unaffected family members. Eur J Haematol 2011;86(5):396–404.
22. Brandefors L, Kimby E, Lundqvist K, et al. Familial Waldenstrom's macroglobulinemia and relation to immune defects, autoimmune diseases, and haematological malignancies – a population-based study from northern Sweden. Acta Oncol 2016;55(1):91–8.
23. Frank C, Fallah M, Chen T, et al. Search for familial clustering of multiple myeloma with any cancer. Leukemia 2016;30:627–32.

24. Vajdic CM, Landgren O, McMaster ML, et al. Medical history, lifestyle, family history, and occupational risk factors for lymphoplasmacytic lymphoma/Waldenström's macroglobulinemia: the InterLymph Non-Hodgkin lymphoma subtypes project. J Natl Cancer Inst Monogr 2014;2014(48):87–97.

25. Treon SP, Hunter ZR, Aggarwal A, et al. Characterization of familial Waldenstrom's macroglobulinemia. Ann Oncol 2006;17(3):488–94.

26. Hanzis C, Ojha RP, Hunter Z, et al. Associated malignancies in patients with Waldenstrom's macroglobulinemia and their kin. Clin Lymphoma Myeloma Leuk 2011;11(1):88–92.

27. Ojha RP, Hanzis CA, Hunter ZR, et al. Family history of non-hematologic cancers among Waldenstrom macroglobulinemia patients: a preliminary study. Cancer Epidemiol 2012;36(3):294–7.

28. Kristinsson SY, Goldin LR, Turesson I, et al. Familial aggregation of lymphoplasmacytic lymphoma/Waldenström macroglobulinemia with solid tumors and myeloid malignancies. Acta Haematol 2012;127:173–7.

29. Custodi P, Cerutti A, Cassani P, et al. Familial occurrence of IgMk gammopathy: no role of HCV infection. Haematologica 1995;80:484–5.

30. Kristinsson SY, Koshiol J, Björkholm M, et al. Immune-related and inflammatory conditions and risk of lymphoplasmacytic lymphoma or Waldenström macroglobulinemia. J Natl Cancer Inst 2010;102(8):557–67.

31. Kyle RA, Therneau TM, Rajkumar SV, et al. Long-term follow-up of IgM monoclonal gammopathy of undetermined significance. Blood 2003;102(10):3759–64.

32. Fine JM, Lambin P, Massari M, et al. Malignant evolution of asymptomatic monoclonal IgM after seven and fifteen years in two siblings of a patient with Waldenström's macroglobulinemia. Acta Med Scand 1982;211:237–9.

33. McMaster ML, Csako G. Protein electrophoresis, Immunoelectrophoresis and immunofixation electrophoresis as predictors for high-risk phenotype in familial Waldenström macroglobulinemia. Int J Cancer 2008;122:1183–8.

34. Kalff MW, Hijmans W. Immunoglobulin analysis in families of macroglobulinaemia patients. Clin Exp Immunol 1969;5(5):479–98.

35. Lock RJ, Unsworth DJ. Immunoglobulins and immunoglobulin subclasses in the elderly. Ann Clin Biochem 2003;40(2):143–8.

36. Crisp HC, Quinn JM. Quantitative immunoglobulins in adulthood. Allergy Asthma Proc 2009;30:649–54.

37. Ögmundsdóttir HM, Sveinsdóttir S, Sigfússon A, et al. Enhanced B cell survival in familial macroglobulinaemia is associated with increased expression of Bcl-2. Clin Exp Immunol 1999;117(2):252–60.

38. Groves FD, Travis LB, Devesa SS, et al. Waldenstrom's macroglobulinemia: incidence patterns in the United States, 1988-1994. Cancer 1998;82(6):1078–81.

39. Elves MW, Brown AK. Cytogenetic studies in a family with Waldenstrom's macroglobuliaemia. J Med Genet 1968;5(2):118–22.

40. McMaster ML, Giambarresi T, Vasquez L, et al. Cytogenetics of familial Waldenström's macroglobulinemia: in pursuit of an understanding of genetic predisposition. Clin Lymphoma 2005;5(4):230–4.

41. Royer RH, Koshiol J, Giambarresi TR, et al. Differential characteristics of Waldenström macroglobulinemia according to patterns of familial aggregation. Blood 2010;115(22):4464–71.

42. Treon SP, Tripsas C, Hanzis C, et al. Familial disease predisposition impacts treatment outcome in patients with Waldenström macroglobulinemia. Clin Lymphoma Myeloma Leuk 2012;12(6):433–7.

43. Steingrímsson V, Lund SH, Turesson I, et al. Population-based study on the impact of the familial form of Waldenström macroglobulinemia on overall survival. Blood 2015;125(13):2174–5.
44. McMaster ML, Goldin LR, Bai Y, et al. Genomewide linkage screen for Waldenström macroglobulinemia susceptibility loci in high-risk families. Am J Hum Genet 2006;79(4):695–701.
45. Liang XS, Caporaso N, McMaster ML, et al. Common genetic variants in candidate genes and risk of familial lymphoid malignancies. Br J Haematol 2009; 146:418–23.
46. Price P, Witt C, Allcock R, et al. The genetic basis for the association of the 8.1 ancestral haplogype (A1, Bi, DR3) with multiple immunopathological diseases. Immunol Rev 1999;167:257–74.
47. Wang SS, Lu Y, Rothman N, et al. Variation in effects of non-Hodgkin lymphoma risk factors according to the human leukocyte antigen (HLA)-DRB1*01:01 allele and ancestral haplotype 8.1. PLoS One 2011;6(11):326949.
48. Abdou AM, Gao X, Cozen W, et al. Human leukocyte antigen (HLA) A1-B8-DR3 (8.1) haplotype, tumor necrosis factor (TNF) G-308A, and risk of non-Hodgkin lymphoma. Leukemia 2010;24(5):1055–88.
49. Grass S, Preuss KD, Wikowicz A, et al. Hyperphosphorylated paratarg-7: a new molecularly defined risk factor for monoclonal gammopathy of undetermined significance of the IgM type and Waldenstrom macroglobulinemia. Blood 2011; 117(10):2918–23.
50. Adamia S, Crainie M, Kriangkum J, et al. Abnormal expression of hyaluronan synthases in patients with Waldenstrom's macroglobulinemia. Semin Oncol 2003; 30(2):165–8.
51. Adamia S, Reichert AA, Kuppusamy H, et al. Inherited and acquired variations in the hyaluronan synthase 1 (HAS1) gene may contribute to disease progression in multiple myeloma and Waldenstrom macroglobulinemia. Blood 2008;112(13):5111–21.
52. Ghosh A, Kuppusamy H, Pilarski LM. Aberrant splice variants of HAS1 (Hyaluronan Synthase 1) multimerize with and modulate normally spliced HAS1 protein: a potential mechanism promoting human cancer. J Biol Chem 2009;284(28): 18840–50.
53. Kuppusamy H, Ögmundsdóttir HM, Baigorri E, et al. Inherited polymorphisms in hyaluronan synthase 1 predict risk of systemic B-cell malignancies but not of breast cancer. PLoS One 2014;9(6):100691.
54. Treon SP, Xu L, Yang G, et al. MYD88 L265P somatic mutation in Waldenström's macroglobulinemia. N Engl J Med 2012;367(9):826–33.
55. Pertesi M, Galia P, Nazaret N, et al. Rare circulating cells in familial Waldenström macroglobulinemia displaying the MYD88 L265P mutation are enriched by Epstein-Barr virus immortalization. PLoS One 2015;10(9):30136515.
56. Roccaro AM, Sacco A, Shi J, et al. Exome sequencing reveals recurrent germ line variants in patients with familial Waldenström macroglobulinemia. Blood 2016; 127(21):2598–606.
57. Jacobs KB, Yeager M, Cullen MG, et al. Realities and limitations of coverage in current "whole"-exome sequencing capture approaches [abstract]. Genet Epidemiol 2010;34(8):919–20.
58. McMaster ML, Goldin LR, Rotunno M, et al. Exploration of rare variants from exome sequencing in families with Waldenström macroglobulinemia [abstract]. In: Proc Amer Assoc Cancer Res 2014. San Diego (CA): April, 2014. p. 1300.
59. Spengler GA, Butler R, Fischer CH, et al. On the question of familial occurrence of paraproteinemia. Helv Med Acta 1966;3:208–19.

60. Linet MS, Humphrey RL, Mehl ES, et al. A case-control and family study of Wal-denstrom's macroglobulinemia. Leukemia 1993;7(9):1363–9.
61. Manschot SM, Notermans NC, van den Berg LH, et al. Three families with poly-neuropathy associated with monoclonal gammopathy. Arch Neurol 2000;57(5): 740–2.
62. Williams RC Jr, Erickson JL, Polesky HF, et al. Studies of monoclonal immuno-globulins (M-components) in various kindreds. Ann Intern Med 1967;67(2): 309–27.
63. Zawadzki ZA, Yoshiharu A, Kraj MA, et al. Familial immunopathies: report of nine families and survey of literature. Cancer 1977;40:2094–101.

Initial Evaluation of the Patient with Waldenström Macroglobulinemia

Jorge J. Castillo, MD*, Steven P. Treon, MD, PhD

KEYWORDS

- Waldenström macroglobulinemia • Bone marrow aspiration • Anemia
- Hyperviscosity • Cryoglobulinemia • Peripheral neuropathy • Bing-Neel syndrome
- Amyloidosis

KEY POINTS

- The initial evaluation of the patient with Waldenström macroglobulinemia can be challenging.
- Not only is Waldenström macroglobulinemia a rare disease, but the clinical features of patients with Waldenström macroglobulinemia can vary greatly from patient to patient.
- The authors provide concise and practical recommendations for the initial evaluation of patients with Waldenström macroglobulinemia, specifically regarding history taking, physical examination, laboratory testing, bone marrow aspiration and biopsy evaluation, and imaging studies.
- The authors review the most common special clinical situations seen in patients with Waldenström macroglobulinemia, especially anemia, hyperviscosity, cryoglobulinemia, peripheral neuropathy, extramedullary disease, Bing-Neel syndrome, and amyloidosis.

INTRODUCTION

Given its rarity and a highly variable clinical presentation, the initial evaluation of the patient with a clinicopathologic diagnosis of Waldenström macroglobulinemia (WM) can be challenging. The clinical manifestations of WM can be associated with infiltration of the bone marrow and other organs by malignant lymphoplasmacytic cells and/or the properties of the monoclonal IgM paraproteinemia, and include anemia, hyperviscosity, extramedullary disease, peripheral neuropathy, cryoglobulinemia, cold agglutinemia, and coagulopathy, among others. It is important to note, however, that a substantial number of patients with WM can be asymptomatic at diagnosis.

Bing Center for Waldenström Macroglobulinemia, Dana-Farber Cancer Institute, Harvard Medical School, 450 Brookline Avenue, Mayer 221, Boston, MA 02215, USA
* Corresponding author.
E-mail address: jorgej_castillo@dfci.harvard.edu

Hematol Oncol Clin N Am 32 (2018) 811–820
https://doi.org/10.1016/j.hoc.2018.05.008
0889-8588/18/© 2018 Elsevier Inc. All rights reserved.

It is paramount to appropriately evaluate patients with WM to better inform the need for further evaluation, appropriateness of treatment initiation, and treatment options. The objective of this review was to succinctly summarize current recommendations with regard to initial evaluation of patients with WM. The recommendations provided herein are in line with those from the International Workshop for Waldenström macroglobulinemia and the National Comprehensive Cancer Network.

ESSENTIAL EVALUATION

The essential evaluation of the patient with a diagnosis of WM must include a history and physical examination, laboratory studies, bone marrow aspiration and biopsy, and computed tomography (CT) scans of the chest, abdomen, and pelvis with intravenous contrast.[1] It is important to note that there is no sign or symptom pathognomonic of WM. However, the presence of particular clinical findings can help to direct additional evaluation. Additionally, other causes of any sign, symptom, or laboratory or imaging finding should be further investigated to determine the likelihood of its relation to WM.

HISTORY

A careful and systematic history taking can provide information not only on the presence of constitutional symptoms such as fevers, night sweats, or unintentional weight loss, but also for potential alternative causes for these symptoms. Symptoms associated with anemia are very common in patients with WM, and include fatigue, malaise, and shortness of breath. Symptomatic hyperviscosity can induce recurrent episodes of spontaneous epistaxis, new-onset headaches, and blurred vision.[2] WM-related neuropathy is typically sensory and affects the feet more than the hands in a bilateral and symmetric pattern. If advanced and prolonged, it can manifest as muscle weakness and muscle wasting.[3] A history of skin color changes induced by exposure to cold temperatures may indicate the presence of cryoglobulins. Recurrent episodes of urticarial rash might be associated with Schnitzler syndrome.[4] Increased bruising or mucosal bleeding can be due to thrombocytopenia or acquired von Willebrand disease. Finally, recurrent upper respiratory infections might indicate secondary hypogammaglobulinemia.

PHYSICAL EXAMINATION

The physical examination can reveal lymphadenopathy and/or hepatosplenomegaly. Raynaud phenomenon or ulcers in the lower extremities or tip of the nose and ears can be manifestations of cryoglobulinemia.[2] Darkening of the urine after exposure to cold might be a manifestation of cold agglutinemia.[5] Skin examination might reveal urticarial rash, lymphomatous lesions, purpura, or bruising. A neurologic examination can reveal sensory or motor deficits in upper and lower extremities and can indicate peripheral neuropathy. Cranial nerve deficits can be a manifestation of Bing-Neel syndrome (BNS).[6] A funduscopic examination can reveal engorgement, increased tortuosity or "sausaging" of retinal vessels or retinal hemorrhages in patients with hyperviscosity.

LABORATORY STUDIES

Essential laboratory studies include a complete blood count, peripheral blood smear evaluation, complete metabolic panel, quantitative serum immunoglobulins (IgA, IgG, and IgM), serum and urine protein electrophoresis with immunofixation and beta-2-microglobulin level. The complete blood count can identify patients with WM with anemia (common), thrombocytopenia (less common), or leukopenia (rare). Other causes of anemia, thrombocytopenia, and leukopenia should be investigated. High serum IgM levels can be associated with artificially low hemoglobin levels owing to volume expansion; transfusions should be avoided in these cases because they could increase serum viscosity.[7] Peripheral blood smear evaluation can show Rouleaux formation and, in rare cases, circulating lymphoplasmacytic cells. The complete metabolic panel can show renal dysfunction, which is rare in patients with WM, but can be associated with amyloidosis, monoclonal immunoglobulin deposition, and lymphoplasmacytic infiltration among others.[8] Rarely, WM can cause hepatic dysfunction. The serum IgM level is used to follow progression of disease or response to therapy and, in some cases, can be associated with a risk of hyperviscosity.[9] Low serum IgA and IgG levels (ie, hypogammaglobulinemia) can be seen in patients with WM at diagnosis.[10] Serum and urine protein electrophoresis with immunofixation will reveal an IgM monoclonal paraprotein, even in cases in whom serum IgM levels are normal. Beta-2-microglobulin levels can be prognostic of survival as a component of the International Prognostic Scoring System for Waldenström macroglobulinemia, along with age, hemoglobin level, platelet count, and serum IgM level.[11]

In special circumstances, additional laboratory testing can be helpful. Cryoglobulins should be obtained in patients with WM with clinical findings of cryoglobulinemia and cold agglutinins in patients with hemolytic anemia triggered by exposure to cold. However, the false-negative ratio of cryoglobulins and cold agglutinins is high, and the diagnosis is frequently made on clinical grounds. Serum viscosity can be measured in patients suspected to have symptomatic hyperviscosity.[12] Screening tests for acquired von Willebrand disease (ie, immunologic assays of von Willebrand factor [VWF], VWF ristocetin cofactor, and factor VIII procoagulant activity) should be obtained in patients suspected to have a bleeding diathesis.[13] Upon response to therapy for WM and with serum IgM levels decreasing, the levels of immunologic assays of VWF, VWF ristocetin cofactor, and factor VIII procoagulant activity do improve and, in many cases, normalize.[13] High levels of immunologic assays of VWF have been associated with worse prognosis in WM.[14] The role of serum free light chain measurements is unclear in WM and is recommended only in cases of suspected light chain amyloidosis. In cases of amyloidosis or monoclonal immunoglobulin deposition with glomerular damage, a 24-hour urine protein quantification might reveal albuminuria.

BONE MARROW ASPIRATION AND BIOPSY

A diagnosis of WM requires, in addition to a monoclonal IgM paraproteinemia, the presence of lymphoplasmacytic lymphoma in the bone marrow or other tissues.[15] A bone marrow aspiration and biopsy with immunophenotyping will help differentiate WM from IgM monoclonal gammopathy of undetermined significance, IgM multiple myeloma (MM) and IgM-secreting lymphomas such as marginal zone lymphoma.[16] The typical appearance of WM includes kappa or lambda light chain-restricted lymphocytes, lymphoplasmacytic cells, and plasma cells.[15] The malignant B-cells express CD19 and CD20 and rarely express CD5, CD10, or CD23, whereas the malignant plasma cells express CD38 or CD138 and show the same restricted light chain expression as the lymphocytic compartment.[17,18] Deletion 6q is the most common cytogenetic abnormality described in WM,[19,20] but it does not seem to have diagnostic or prognostic value. The bone marrow aspirate should be evaluated for the MYD88 L265P mutation, which is present in 90% to 95% of patients with WM,[21] and can help to further differentiate WM from other conditions. The MYD88 L265P mutation has also been described in 50% to 80% of individuals with IgM monoclonal gammopathy of undetermined significance and in 5% to 10% of patients with marginal zone lymphoma, but not in patients with MM.[22,23] Therefore, the sole presence of the MYD88 L265P mutation is not diagnostic of WM. In contrast, the absence of MYD88 L265P mutation should not exclude the diagnosis of WM. About 5% to 10% of patients with WM will not have a MYD88 mutation, but would still meet the clinicopathologic criteria for WM and should be treated as such. Patients without MYD88 mutations have a worse outcome and have a higher risk for transformation to diffuse large B-cell lymphoma.[24] Rare cases of non-L265P MYD88 mutations have been described (approximately 2%), and should be managed as patients with MYD88 L265P mutation.[25] In about 40% of patients with WM, somatic mutations in the CXCR4 gene have been described.[26–28] Patients with WM with CXCR4 mutations tend to present with higher serum IgM levels, lower rates of extramedullary disease, and higher rates of hyperviscosity and acquired von Willebrand disease.[9,13] The presence of CXCR4 mutations have been associated with a longer time to response, lower rates of deep responses, and shorter response duration when treated with the oral BTK inhibitor ibrutinib.[29] CXCR4 mutations can also impact time to response and depth of response to ixazomib.[30] Testing for non-L265P mutations and CXCR4 mutations are not standard and not available in most laboratories.

COMPUTED TOMOGRAPHY SCANS

CT scans of the chest, abdomen, and pelvis with intravenous contrast are essential in patients with WM with suspected extramedullary disease, such as lymphadenopathy, hepatosplenomegaly, or pleural effusions, or in patients being considered for treatment initiation. If extramedullary disease is present, CT scans during and/or after treatment are advised to assess response. CT scans can be useful when differentiating an IgM flare from disease progression in patients treated with rituximab-containing regimens.[31,32] The role of PET/CT in WM is not well-established; however, it could be helpful in rare cases suspicious of transformation to diffuse large B-cell lymphoma, which can be seen in 2% to 3% of patients with WM.[33] In this context, areas of significantly higher 18F-fludeoxyglucose avidity are suspicious for aggressive transformation or other malignancies and should be biopsied accordingly.

SPECIAL SITUATIONS

This section provides guidance on the evaluation of special situations, specifically anemia, hyperviscosity and cryoglobulinemia, peripheral neuropathy, extramedullary disease and BNS, and amyloidosis.

ANEMIA

Anemia is the most common reason to initiate therapy in patients with WM. Anemia in patients with WM can be due to bone marrow replacement by the disease, iron deficiency, and/or hemolysis. In anemic patients with WM in whom the bone marrow burden of disease is low, another cause of anemia should be specifically sought. Iron studies (ie, iron, total iron-binding capacity, and ferritin) should be performed in all cases. In patients with absolute iron deficiency (low iron saturation and low ferritin level), gastrointestinal blood loss should be evaluated with upper, lower, and capsule (small bowel) endoscopies. In some patients, there can be evidence of functional iron deficiency (low iron saturation and normal/high ferritin level). WM cells can produce hepcidin, which is a regulator of serum iron content, inducing a mixture of absolute and functional iron deficiency.[34] In these cases, as long as there is no other criterion to treat, intravenous iron supplementation can improve the anemia and delay WM-directed treatment.[35] Rarely, anemia can be secondary to hemolysis. In these patients, a hemolytic panel including reticulocyte counts, lactate dehydrogenase, haptoglobin, direct Coombs test, and cold agglutinins should be performed. In patients with severe cold agglutinemia, plasmapheresis should be started promptly to remove cold agglutinins. Other causes of anemia such as cobalamin and folate deficiency; renal, hepatic, or thyroid dysfunction; nonautoimmune hemolysis (eg, hemoglobinopathies); or other primary bone marrow processes should be ruled out.

HYPERVISCOSITY AND CRYOGLOBULINEMIA

Symptomatic hyperviscosity owing to high serum IgM levels can complicate the course of WM in 10% to 15% of patients and can have deleterious effects on the vision and neurologic function of patients.[9] The most common symptoms associated with hyperviscosity include recurrent spontaneous nosebleeds, headaches, blurred vision that does not correct with glasses, tinnitus, vertigo, and slow mentation.[12] Symptomatic hyperviscosity is rarely seen in patients with serum IgM levels of less than 3000 mg/dL.[9] In patients with serum IgM levels of 3000 or greater, obtaining serum viscosity and cryoglobulins can be helpful. Some patients are symptomatic at viscosity levels of 4 cP and most at 6 cP. A funduscopic examination must also be performed to evaluate for hyperviscosity-related changes in the retinal vessels, which can occur in asymptomatic patients. Patients with a serum IgM of 6000 mg/dL or greater have a median time to symptomatic hyperviscosity of 3 months and should be considered for therapy.[9] Plasmapheresis should be initiated promptly in patients with WM with signs and symptoms of hyperviscosity. Plasmapheresis, however, should be used only temporarily until definitive therapy for WM is instituted.[36] The most common manifestations of cryoglobulinemia include acrocyanosis, palpable purpura, livedo reticularis, nonhealing ulcers on the lower extremities, and discoloration of the tip of the nose and ears upon exposure to cold temperatures. Type I cryoglobulinemia is usually associated with WM, and type II is associated with hepatitis C infection. The presence of cryoglobulins can aggravate serum viscosity and should be evaluated while blood samples are at 37°C to prevent precipitation, which in turn can give falsely low IgM level and false-negative results.[2] Plasmapheresis will promptly remove cryoglobulins and provide symptomatic relief in these patients. Blood warmers might be needed in these patients to prevent cryoglobulin precipitation during plasmapheresis.[7]

PERIPHERAL NEUROPATHY

About 20% of patients with WM can present with symptoms of peripheral neuropathy. The most common clinical presentation of WM-related neuropathy is a sensory neuropathy characterized by a slowly progressing bilateral and symmetric numbness of the lower extremities. Nerve conduction studies typically show a demyelinating pattern.[3] In a portion of patients, antimyelin-associated globulin antibodies can be detected and would support the diagnosis.[37] In patients with atypical neuropathic symptoms or axonal patterns in nerve conduction studies, other causes of neuropathy should be evaluated. These include radiculopathy, diabetes, cobalamin deficiency, thyroid dysfunction, human immunodeficiency virus infection, Lyme disease, syphilis, autoimmune conditions (eg, lupus, vasculitis, or chronic inflammatory demyelinating polyneuropathy), and BNS. It is important to note that prolonged demyelination (ie, years) can induce axonal damage. In some cases, WM-related neuropathy may be due to lymphoplasmacytic infiltration of the nerve fibers, cryoglobulinemia, or amyloidosis. Nerve conduction studies and additional testing (ie, cryoglobulins, free light chain levels, or nerve biopsy) might be needed to investigate these further. Nerve biopsies should not be performed routinely, because they can cause permanent neurologic deficits.[38]

EXTRAMEDULLARY DISEASE AND BING-NEEL SYNDROME

Extramedullary disease can be detected in 20% of patients with WM at diagnosis but it can be seen in up to 60% of patients at relapse. The most common sites of extramedullary disease are the lymph nodes and the spleen. Rarely, WM can affect kidneys, pleura, skeletal bone, and central nervous system. CT scans are helpful not only in identifying extramedullary disease, but also in assessing response on extramedullary sites during and after therapy. Based on CT criteria, lymph nodes above the diaphragm are considered pathologic if greater than 1.5 cm in longest diameter, whereas lymph nodes below the diaphragm are pathologic if greater than 2.0 cm. A spleen size of greater than 15.0 cm establishes splenomegaly. However, the sole presence of pathologic lymph nodes and/or splenomegaly does not constitute a criterion to initiate therapy, because they would have to be symptomatic.[39] In cases of extramedullary involvement of rare sites, a biopsy could be indicated to establish the diagnosis. Renal involvement has been reported in up to 3% of patients with WM, and can be due to amyloidosis, monoclonal IgM or free light chain deposition, light chain cast nephropathy, or lymphoplasmacytic cell infiltration, among others.[8] In patients with WM with renal involvement, monoclonal IgM deposition, and lymphoplasmacytic infiltration respond better to therapy than light chain cast nephropathy or amyloidosis. Pleural effusions are rare in patients with WM. A thoracentesis is needed to evaluate the effusion for the presence of malignant cells. The fluid should be sent for cytology, flow cytometry and polymerase chain reaction assays for IgH gene rearrangement and MYD88 L265P mutation. In some cases, the lymphoplasmacytic cells are adhered to pleural fenestrations and might not be readily identifiable by cytology or flow cytometry. In these cases, the diagnosis can be supported by the detection of IgH gene rearrangement or the MYD88 L265P mutation by polymerase chain reaction.[40] Lytic bone lesions, although common in MM, are rare in WM. Lytic bone lesions can also be due to other malignant processes, and a biopsy is advisable for proper diagnosis. The management of lytic bone lesions associated with WM should mimic the management of MM.

BNS is a rare complication of WM seen in about 1% of cases and refers to the involvement of the central nervous system by lymphoplasmacytic cells.[6] The most common manifestations of BNS include motor deficits, cranial nerve palsies, altered mental status, seizures, headaches, and atypical neuropathic symptoms.[41,42] BNS can occur at any time during the course of the disease. BNS can be the presenting symptom of WM and can also be diagnosed when in apparent complete systemic response to therapy. The evaluation of patients suspected of having BNS should include MRI studies with gadolinium enhancement of the brain and spine and a lumbar puncture for cerebrospinal fluid analysis. In most cases, the MRI shows leptomeningeal enhancement. Intraparenchymal brain lesions can be seen in a minority of cases. The cerebrospinal fluid should be sent for cytology, flow cytometry, and polymerase chain reaction assays for IgH gene rearrangement and MYD88 L265P mutation. A brain biopsy can be performed in patients with brain lesions without cerebrospinal fluid involvement. Treatment options for BNS are limited to agents with good central nervous system penetration such as methotrexate, fludarabine, bendamustine, and ibrutinib.[43]

AMYLOIDOSIS

Amyloidosis is a rare complication of WM caused by the aggregation of misfolded proteins that deposit as fibrils in several organs, including the kidneys, heart, peripheral nerves, liver, and gastrointestinal tract. Of the several types of amyloidosis, the most commonly associated with WM is light chain (AL) amyloidosis.[44] Rare cases of IgM-related heavy chain (AH) and heavy and light chain (ALH) amyloidosis have been described in patients with WM. In patients suspected to have amyloidosis, a fat pad biopsy and/or bone marrow biopsy material should be stained with Congo red; amyloid produces a characteristic apple-green birefringence on microscopic examination under polarized light. In cases in which both fat pad and bone marrow evaluations are negative for amyloid, but a strong suspicion remains, a biopsy of the affected organ is advisable.[1] Amyloid typing is recommended in most cases and should be performed using mass spectrometry.[45,46] Immunoelectron microscopy or immunohistochemistry may also be used for this purpose.[47,48] Renal involvement by amyloid should be investigated with a 24-hour urine protein measurement and serum free light chain levels, which can be used for response assessment. Cardiac involvement should be evaluated by obtaining troponin or brain natriuretic peptide levels, which have prognostic implications. The MYD88 L265P mutation has been detected in more than 70% of patients with IgM-related amyloidosis.[49] The prognosis of patients with IgM-related AL amyloidosis might be more favorable than those with AL amyloidosis.[50]

SUMMARY

The initial evaluation of the patient with a diagnosis of WM can be challenging, but the thoughtful application of relevant data from the history, physical examination, laboratory tests, bone marrow aspiration and biopsy, and imaging studies can provide valuable insights for the management of these patients.

REFERENCES

1. Castillo JJ, Garcia-Sanz R, Hatjiharissi E, et al. Recommendations for the diagnosis and initial evaluation of patients with Waldenstrom macroglobulinaemia: a task force from the 8th International Workshop on Waldenstrom Macroglobulinaemia. Br J Haematol 2016;175:77–86.
2. Stone MJ. Waldenstrom's macroglobulinemia: hyperviscosity syndrome and cryoglobulinemia. Clin Lymphoma Myeloma 2009;9:97–9.
3. Baehring JM, Hochberg EP, Raje N, et al. Neurological manifestations of Waldenstrom macroglobulinemia. Nat Clin Pract Neurol 2008;4:547–56.
4. Schnitzler L, Schubert B, Boasson M, et al. Urticaire chronique, lésions osseuses, macroglobulinémie IgM: maladie de Waldenström ? 2ème présentation. Bull Soc Fr Dermatol Syphiligr 1974;81:363.
5. Berentsen S. Cold agglutinin-mediated autoimmune hemolytic anemia in Waldenstrom's macroglobulinemia. Clin Lymphoma Myeloma 2009;9:110–2.
6. Bing J, Neel A. Two cases of hyperglobulinemia with affection of the central nervous system on a toxi-infectious basis. Acta Med Scand 1936;LXXXVIII:492–506.
7. Treon SP. How I treat Waldenstrom macroglobulinemia. Blood 2009;114:2375–85.
8. Vos JM, Gustine J, Rennke HG, et al. Renal disease related to Waldenstrom macroglobulinaemia: incidence, pathology and clinical outcomes. Br J Haematol 2016;175:623–30.
9. Gustine JN, Meid K, Dubeau T, et al. Serum IgM level as predictor of symptomatic hyperviscosity in patients with Waldenstrom macroglobulinaemia. Br J Haematol 2017;177:717–25.
10. Hunter ZR, Manning RJ, Hanzis C, et al. IgA and IgG hypogammaglobulinemia in Waldenstrom's macroglobulinemia. Haematologica 2010;95:470–5.

11. Morel P, Duhamel A, Gobbi P, et al. International prognostic scoring system for Waldenstrom macroglobulinemia. Blood 2009;113:4163–70.

12. Stone MJ, Bogen SA. Evidence-based focused review of management of hyperviscosity syndrome. Blood 2012;119:2205–8.

13. Castillo JJ, Gustine J, Meid K, et al. Low levels of von Willebrand markers associate with high serum IgM levels, and improve with response to therapy, in patients with Waldenstrom Macroglobulinemia. Br J Haematol 2018. [Epub ahead of print].

14. Hivert B, Caron C, Petit S, et al. Clinical and prognostic implications of low or high level of von Willebrand factor in patients with Waldenstrom macroglobulinemia. Blood 2012;120:3214–21.

15. Swerdlow SH, Berger F, Pileri SA, et al. Lymphoplasmacytic lymphoma. In: Swerdlow SH, Campo E, Harris NL, et al, editors. WHO classification of tumours of haematopoietic and lymphoid tissues. Lyon (France): IARC; 2008. p. 194–5.

16. Castillo JJ, Treon SP. Toward personalized treatment in Waldenstrom macroglobulinemia. Hematology Am Soc Hematol Educ Program 2017;2017:365–70.

17. Konoplev S, Medeiros LJ, Bueso-Ramos CE, et al. Immunophenotypic profile of lymphoplasmacytic lymphoma/Waldenstrom macroglobulinemia. Am J Clin Pathol 2005;124:414–20.

18. Paiva B, Montes MC, Garcia-Sanz R, et al. Multiparameter flow cytometry for the identification of the Waldenstrom's clone in IgM-MGUS and Waldenstrom's Macroglobulinemia: new criteria for differential diagnosis and risk stratification. Leukemia 2014;28:166–73.

19. Braggio E, Fonseca R. Genomic abnormalities of Waldenstrom macroglobulinemia and related low-grade B-cell lymphomas. Clin Lymphoma Myeloma Leuk 2013;13:198–201.

20. Nguyen-Khac F, Lambert J, Chapiro E, et al. Chromosomal aberrations and their prognostic value in a series of 174 untreated patients with Waldenstrom's macroglobulinemia. Haematologica 2013;98:649–54.

21. Treon SP, Xu L, Yang G, et al. MYD88 L265P somatic mutation in Waldenstrom's macroglobulinemia. N Engl J Med 2012;367:826–33.

22. Jimenez C, Sebastian E, Chillon MC, et al. MYD88 L265P is a marker highly characteristic of, but not restricted to, Waldenstrom's macroglobulinemia. Leukemia 2013;27:1722–8.

23. Poulain S, Roumier C, Decambron A, et al. MYD88 L265P mutation in Waldenstrom macroglobulinemia. Blood 2013;121:4504–11.

24. Treon SP, Gustine J, Xu L, et al. MYD88 wild-type Waldenstrom Macroglobulinaemia: differential diagnosis, risk of histological transformation, and overall survival. Br J Haematol 2018;180:374–80.

25. Treon SP, Xu L, Hunter Z. MYD88 mutations and response to ibrutinib in Waldenstrom's macroglobulinemia. N Engl J Med 2015;373:584–6.

26. Hunter ZR, Xu L, Yang G, et al. The genomic landscape of Waldenstrom macroglobulinemia is characterized by highly recurring MYD88 and WHIM-like CXCR4 mutations, and small somatic deletions associated with B-cell lymphomagenesis. Blood 2014;123:1637–46.

27. Poulain S, Roumier C, Venet-Caillault A, et al. Genomic landscape of CXCR4 mutations in Waldenstrom macroglobulinemia. Clin Cancer Res 2016;22:1480–8.

28. Schmidt J, Federmann B, Schindler N, et al. MYD88 L265P and CXCR4 mutations in lymphoplasmacytic lymphoma identify cases with high disease activity. Br J Haematol 2015;169:795–803.

29. Treon SP, Meid K, Gustine J, et al. Long-term follow-up of previously treated patients who received ibrutinib for symptomatic Waldenstrom's macroglobulinemia: update of pivotal clinical trial. Blood 2017;130:2766.
30. Castillo JJ, Gustine J, Meid K, et al. Ixazomib, dexamethasone and rituximab in previously untreated patients with Waldenström macroglobulinemia. Blood 2016;128:2956.
31. Ghobrial IM, Fonseca R, Greipp PR, et al. Initial immunoglobulin M 'flare' after rituximab therapy in patients diagnosed with Waldenstrom macroglobulinemia: an Eastern Cooperative Oncology Group Study. Cancer 2004;101:2593–8.
32. Treon SP, Branagan AR, Hunter Z, et al. Paradoxical increases in serum IgM and viscosity levels following rituximab in Waldenstrom's macroglobulinemia. Ann Oncol 2004;15:1481–3.
33. Castillo JJ, Gustine J, Meid K, et al. Histological transformation to diffuse large B-cell lymphoma in patients with Waldenstrom macroglobulinemia. Am J Hematol 2016;91:1032–5.
34. Ciccarelli BT, Patterson CJ, Hunter ZR, et al. Hepcidin is produced by lymphoplasmacytic cells and is associated with anemia in Waldenstrom's macroglobulinemia. Clin Lymphoma Myeloma Leuk 2011;11:160–3.
35. Treon SP, Tripsas CK, Ciccarelli BT, et al. Patients with Waldenstrom macroglobulinemia commonly present with iron deficiency and those with severely depressed transferrin saturation levels show response to parenteral iron administration. Clin Lymphoma Myeloma Leuk 2013;13:241–3.
36. Leblond V, Kastritis E, Advani R, et al. Treatment recommendations from the Eighth International Workshop on Waldenstrom's Macroglobulinemia. Blood 2016;128:1321–8.
37. Levine T, Pestronk A, Florence J, et al. Peripheral neuropathies in Waldenstrom's macroglobulinaemia. J Neurol Neurosurg Psychiatry 2006;77:224–8.
38. D'Sa S, Kersten MJ, Castillo JJ, et al. Investigation and management of IgM and Waldenstrom-associated peripheral neuropathies: recommendations from the IWWM-8 consensus panel. Br J Haematol 2017;176:728–42.
39. Kyle RA, Treon SP, Alexanian R, et al. Prognostic markers and criteria to initiate therapy in Waldenstrom's macroglobulinemia: consensus panel recommendations from the Second International Workshop on Waldenstrom's Macroglobulinemia. Semin Oncol 2003;30:116–20.
40. Gustine JN, Meid K, Hunter ZR, et al. MYD88 mutations can be used to identify malignant pleural effusions in Waldenstrom macroglobulinaemia. Br J Haematol 2018;180:578–81.
41. Castillo JJ, D'Sa S, Lunn MP, et al. Central nervous system involvement by Waldenstrom macroglobulinaemia (Bing-Neel syndrome): a multi-institutional retrospective study. Br J Haematol 2016;172:709–15.
42. Simon L, Fitsiori A, Lemal R, et al. Bing-Neel syndrome, a rare complication of Waldenstrom macroglobulinemia: analysis of 44 cases and review of the literature. A study on behalf of the French Innovative Leukemia Organization (FILO). Haematologica 2015;100:1587–94.
43. Minnema MC, Kimby E, D'Sa S, et al. Guideline for the diagnosis, treatment and response criteria for Bing-Neel syndrome. Haematologica 2017;102:43–51.
44. Sipe JD, Benson MD, Buxbaum JN, et al. Nomenclature 2014: amyloid fibril proteins and clinical classification of the amyloidosis. Amyloid 2014;21:221–4.
45. Brambilla F, Lavatelli F, Valentini V, et al. Changes in tissue proteome associated with ATTR amyloidosis: insights into pathogenesis. Amyloid 2012;19(Suppl 1):11–3.

46. Vrana JA, Gamez JD, Madden BJ, et al. Classification of amyloidosis by laser microdissection and mass spectrometry-based proteomic analysis in clinical biopsy specimens. Blood 2009;114:4957–9.
47. Fernandez de Larrea C, Verga L, Morbini P, et al. A practical approach to the diagnosis of systemic amyloidoses. Blood 2015;125:2239–44.
48. Schonland SO, Hegenbart U, Bochtler T, et al. Immunohistochemistry in the classification of systemic forms of amyloidosis: a systematic investigation of 117 patients. Blood 2012;119:488–93.
49. Chakraborty R, Novak AJ, Ansell SM, et al. First report of MYD88(L265P) somatic mutation in IgM-associated light chain amyloidosis. Amyloid 2017;24:42–3.
50. Sissoko M, Sanchorawala V, Seldin D, et al. Clinical presentation and treatment responses in IgM-related AL amyloidosis. Amyloid 2015;22:229–35.

Alkylating Agents in the Treatment of Waldenström Macroglobulinemia

Christian Buske, MD

KEYWORDS

- Alkylating agents • Waldenström macroglobulinemia • DRC • CHOP
- Bendamustine

KEY POINTS

- Chemotherapy in combination with rituximab is still a key treatment element in Waldenström macroglobulinemia (WM).
- Among chemotherapeutics, alkylating agents are still widely used in WM.
- The combination of dexamethasone, cyclophosphamide, and rituximab is a highly active treatment option with a favorable toxicity profile.
- Future studies must define the role of alkylating agents in the treatment of WM in the era of emerging chemotherapy-free targeted therapies.

INTRODUCTION

In recent years, the emergence of ibrutinib has dramatically changed the treatment landscape of Waldenström macroglobulinemia (WM), underlining that chemotherapy-free therapy has an immense potential in this disease. In fact, ibrutinib is the most powerful single agent in WM treatment.[1] However, ibrutinib treatment has its limitations and challenges. There is genotype-dependent sensitivity toward ibrutinib with inferior response rates in patients with mutations of CXCR4 or wildtype MYD88 and wildtype CXCR4 genes.[2] In addition, ibrutinib has to be given until progression and, therefore, is a permanent therapy, causing substantial treatment costs. Furthermore, in Europe, ibrutinib is only approved in patients not eligible for chemoimmunotherapy. Based on all this, chemotherapy in combination with rituximab is still a cornerstone in the treatment of WM, reflected by recommendations in international and national guidelines.[3,4] Among the different chemotherapeutics, alkylating agents are the most important, particularly when bendamustine, which carries the characteristics of both an alkyl and a purine analogue, is added. Purine analogues, such as

Comprehensive Cancer Center Ulm, Institute of Experimental Cancer Research, University Hospital Ulm, Albert-Einstein-Allee 11, Ulm 89081, Germany
E-mail address: christian.buske@uni-ulm.de

Hematol Oncol Clin N Am 32 (2018) 821–827
https://doi.org/10.1016/j.hoc.2018.05.009
0889-8588/18/© 2018 Elsevier Inc. All rights reserved.

fludarabine, are highly efficient drugs in WM but have lost popularity because they can induce considerable toxicity by immunosuppression and myelotoxicity.[5] This article summarizes treatment outcomes for alkylating agents in WM.

RITUXIMAB, CYCLOPHOSPHAMIDE, DOXORUBICIN, VINCRISTINE, AND PREDNISONE

Rituximab, cyclophosphamide, doxorubicin, vincristine, and prednisone (R-CHOP) was developed more than 40 years ago and is still the backbone of treatment of different lymphoma entities, such as diffuse large cell lymphoma or follicular lymphoma. In WM, this combination regimen is highly effective, as documented in independent prospective trials. In a prospective randomized trial, the German Low-Grade Lymphoma Study Group could demonstrate that R-CHOP is a well-tolerated and effective treatment for first-line treatment of WM.[6] In the study, 48 WM subjects were randomly assigned to R-CHOP (n = 23) or cyclophosphamide, doxorubicin, vincristine, and prednisone (CHOP) (n = 25). In the R-CHOP arm, a significantly higher overall response rate (ORR) of 91% versus 60% for CHOP alone was observed (P = .0188), whereas the complete remission (CR) rates were not statistically different (9% vs 4%; P = .60). R-CHOP led to a significantly longer time-to-treatment failure, with a median 63 months for R-CHOP versus 22 months in the CHOP arm (P = .0241) (**Fig. 1**). The Eastern Cooperative Oncology Group trial reported about its experience with the R-CHOP combination in the same setting: 91% of the subjects achieved objective response (PR) with a rapid median time to response of 1.6 months; at that time, with a median follow-up time of 18.3 months, median duration of response (DR) had not been reached. Myelosuppression was the main toxicity.[7] These studies indicate that combinations of rituximab with CHOP are highly effective and well-tolerated in medically fit patients. In particular, younger patients, in whom stem cell collection for later myeloablative treatment approaches is considered, R-CHOP is an excellent regimen. However, in many patients, particularly the elderly, R-CHOP is considered too toxic because of its myelosuppressive effects. Also, there is concern about applying neurotoxic vincristine to patients suffering from a disease that often causes neuropathy.

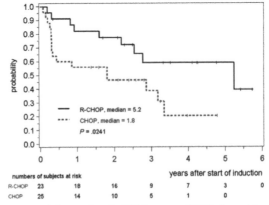

Fig. 1. Time-to-treatment failure after R-CHOP versus CHOP for subjects with treatment-naïve WM. (*Adapted from* Buske C, Hoster E, Dreyling M, et al. The addition of rituximab to front-line therapy with CHOP (R-CHOP) results in a higher response rate and longer time to treatment failure in patients with lymphoplasmacytic lymphoma: results of a randomized trial of the German Low-Grade Lymphoma Study Group (GLSG). Leukemia 2009;23(1):158; with permission.)

DEXAMETHASONE, RITUXIMAB, AND CYCLOPHOSPHAMIDE

Dimopoulos and colleagues[8,9] introduced a very interesting regimen consisting of dexamethasone, rituximab, and cyclophosphamide (DRC). The schedule was 20 mg dexamethasone followed by 375 mg/m^2 rituximab intravenously on day 1 and 100 mg/m^2 cyclophosphamide orally twice a day on days 1 to 5. This regimen was highly effective in a phase II trial in 72 previously untreated subjects with symptomatic WM. An objective response was documented in 83% of subjects, including 7% with CR and 67% with partial remission (PR). Furthermore, the median time to response was 4.1 months. The 2-year progression-free survival (PFS) rate for the total subject group was 67% and for responding subjects 80% (**Fig. 2**). This remarkable activity was paralleled by only moderate myelotoxicity, with only 9% of subjects experiencing grade 3 or 4 neutropenia and none experiencing grade 3 or 4 thrombocytopenia. The final analysis of this trial confirmed the high activity of this immunochemotherapy paralleled by a favorable toxicity profile.[10]

CHLORAMBUCIL

Chlorambucil has been used for more than 4 decades in the treatment of indolent lymphoma. Chlorambucil was and is still used, particularly in elderly patients with WM.

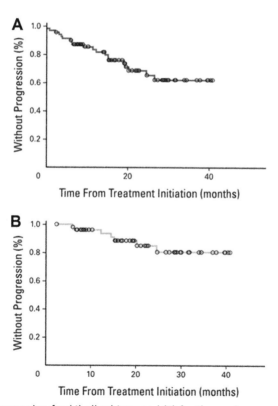

Fig. 2. Time to progression for (A) all subjects and (B) for those who responded to first-line treatment with DRC. (*From* Dimopoulos MA, Anagnostopoulos A, Kyrtsonis MC, et al. Primary treatment of Waldenström macroglobulinemia with dexamethasone, rituximab, and cyclophosphamide. J Clin Oncol 2007;25(22):3346; with permission.)

However, response rates and the DR are inferior to those achieved with rituximab and polychemotherapy combinations. The randomized WM1 study, a large multinational trial, enrolled 339 subjects with treatment-naïve WM and randomized them between chlorambucil and fludarabine. The primary endpoint was ORR. With chlorambucil, the ORR was 38.6% compared with 47.8% in the fludarabine arm ($P = .07$). With a median follow-up of 36 months, the median PFS and DR was 27.1 months and 19.9 months for chlorambucil compared with 36.3 months ($P = .012$) and 38.3 months ($P<.001$) for fludarabine, respectively. However, grade 3 to 4 neutropenia was significantly higher in subjects treated with fludarabine (36%) compared with subjects treated with chlorambucil (17.8%; $P<.001$), whereas the rate of second malignancies were significantly more frequent in the chlorambucil arm, with a 6-year cumulative incidence rate of 20.6% versus 3.7% in the fludarabine arm ($P = .001$). These data demonstrate that chlorambucil has anti-WM activity but significantly lower than that described for the combinations of R-CHOP or DRC. In addition, chlorambucil showed long-term toxicity with a comparatively high rate of second malignancies, including solid cancer, as well as secondary hematological neoplasms, such as 3 cases of myelodysplastic syndrome. Data for the efficacy of chlorambucil in combination with rituximab unfortunately do not exist. However, it is doubtful whether therapies based on chlorambucil will be able to compete with less toxic chemoimmunotherapies or chemotherapy-free approaches, such as ibrutinib.

BENDAMUSTINE-RITUXIMAB

Bendamustine is a chemotherapeutic drug that chemically displays characteristics of both of a purine nucleoside analogue and an alkylating agent. Developed in the 1960s, in postwar communist East Germany, as a competitor to established alkylating drugs, such as cyclophosphamide, it has experienced a rebirth based on its high efficacy in follicular lymphoma and its favorable toxicity profile. This rediscovery was primarily based on a multicenter, randomized, open-label, noninferiority German trial that randomized subjects with newly diagnosed stage III or IV indolent or mantle-cell lymphoma between R-CHOP and bendamustine-rituximab (B-R), in which 90 mg/m^2 bendamustine was given on days 1 and 2 of a 4-week cycle for a maximum of 6 cycles. The primary endpoint was PFS, with a noninferiority margin of 10%. Of the subjects, 274 were assigned to B-R (261 assessed) and 275 to R-CHOP (253 assessed). At a median follow-up of 45 months, median PFS was significantly longer in the B-R arm compared with the R-CHOP group, with 69.5 versus 31.2 months (hazard ratio 0.58; $P<.0001$). B-R had a different toxicity profile than R-CHOP, with lower rates of alopecia and less myelotoxicity, infections, and peripheral neuropathy. A subgroup analysis comprising 41 evaluable subjects with WM documented high response rates in both arms, with 96% for B-R and 94% for R-CHOP. Both treatments were not able to induce CRs. However, the median PFS was longer for B-R, with a median of 69.5 versus 28.1 months for R-CHOP after a median follow-up of 46 months for the total subject population (**Fig. 3**).[11] Although this was a subgroup analysis with a limited number of subjects, these early results pointed to a remarkable activity of B-R in WM and indicated that B-R is another highly attractive treatment option in this often elderly group of patients. Recently, the first results of a subgroup analysis of a prospective randomized trial testing the efficacy of maintenance versus observation after B-R induction were presented. Treatment-naïve WM subjects received a maximum of 6 cycles of B-R. Responding subjects (at least achieving a PR) were eligible for further treatment and were randomized to observation or 2 years of rituximab maintenance every 2 months. The primary endpoint was PFS. Of the subjects, 162 had newly diagnosed

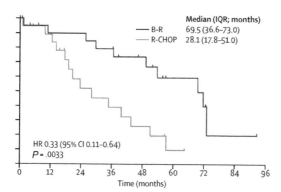

Fig. 3. PFS after B-R versus R-CHOP as first-line treatment in WM subjects. (*From* Rummel MJ, Niederle N, Maschmeyer G, et al. Bendamustine plus rituximab versus CHOP plus rituximab as first-line treatment for patients with indolent and mantle-cell lymphomas: an open-label, multicentre, randomised, phase 3 non-inferiority trial. Lancet 2013;381(9873):1206; Reprinted with permission from Elsevier.)

WM. At the time of analysis, 116 subjects were evaluable for response, with an ORR of 86%, confirming that WM treatment with B-R is highly effective.[12] Data for the maintenance phase have not been presented to date. In a phase II study, the outcome of 30 relapsed or refractory WM subjects after bendamustine-containing therapy was reported. Subjects received B-R (24 subjects) or ofatumumab with bendamustine in the case of rituximab intolerance. The median number of treatment cycles was 5. The ORR was 83.3%, with 5 subjects achieving very good PR and 20 achieving PR. The median estimated PFS for all subjects was 13 months. There were cases of prolonged myelosuppression in subjects who had received prior nucleoside analogues.[13]

SUMMARY

Taken together, the data demonstrate that chemotherapy in combination with rituximab is a highly effective therapy with manageable toxicity in patients with WM. In particular, DRC and B-R are widely used regimens in this disease because of their efficacy and favorable toxicity profile, which has been documented in independent prospective clinical trials. However, recent data on the safety of B-R in the large international randomized Gallium study, which included more than 1000 treatment-naïve subjects with advanced stage follicular lymphoma and 200 subjects with different subtypes of marginal zone lymphoma, showed an unexpected high rate of treatment mortality, reaching higher than 10% in marginal zone lymphoma.[14,15] Most of the treatment-associated deaths were caused by fatal infections, probably due to the prolonged T-cell suppression caused by bendamustine. This stood in clear contrast to R-CHOP, which could be also selected as induction treatment in this trial. Assuredly, WM is a different biological disease than follicular lymphoma or marginal zone lymphoma. In addition, in the Gallium trial, B-R was followed by rituximab maintenance, which might have contributed to the observed toxicity. Rituximab maintenance is more uncommon in WM compared with follicular lymphoma based on the lack of prospective data. Nevertheless, in patients with high risk for infections, bendamustine should be used with caution, and antibacterial (against *Pneumocystis jiroveci* pneumonia) and antiviral (against cytomegalovirus) prophylaxis should be considered. In that respect, DRC is a valid treatment alternative. A recent retrospective comparison between B-R and DRC of 160 consecutive subjects treated in routine clinical practice reported on the efficacy of the 2 regimens: 60 subjects were treated with B-R, 100 subjects with DRC. From the 60 B-R and 100 DRC subjects, 43 and 50 subjects had relapsed or refractory WM, respectively. Subjects' MYD88L265P mutation status was available. For treatment-naïve subjects, the ORR was comparable with 93% and 96% for B-R and DRC, respectively (P = .55). However, there was a trend toward a difference for the 2-year PFS with B-R and DRC having 88% and 61%, respectively (P = .07). For relapsed subjects, there was a trend toward a higher response rate and a prolonged PFS when treated with B-R (ORR 95% with B-R vs 87% with DRC, P = .45; median PFS with B-R 58 vs 32 months with DRC, 2-year PFS with B-R 66% vs 53% with DRC; P = .08). The same trend was also observed for the median disease-specific survival, which was not reached with B-R compared with 166 months with DRC (P = .51). These data demonstrate that B-R has a somewhat higher efficacy compared with DRC, which is, however, associated with higher toxicity, as demonstrated in the prospective clinical trials previously mentioned. Of note, the time-to-event endpoints and depth of response were independent of the MYD88 mutation status in this study, indicating that the activity of both regimens is not compromised by the subjects' MYD88 mutation status.[16] This superiority in efficacy was confirmed in another retrospective study, which compared outcomes between the 2 regimens in WM subjects, partly receiving rituximab maintenance after induction. This study included 57 and 38 subjects treated with B-R and DRC, respectively. The median time to best response was shorter for B-R compared with DRC (18 vs 30 months, respectively) and B-R was associated with better median PFS than DRC (5.5 vs 4.8 years, respectively). Importantly, the 10-year overall survival rate was also higher for B-R group (95% compared with 81%, respectively).[17] Despite this trend to more efficacy for B-R, data should be interpreted with caution due to the retrospective nature of the data. Both regimens should be considered as standard treatment option in WM and treatment should be selected according to the individual patient's characteristics; for instance, the presence of comorbidities or need for a rapid lymphoma response.

The key question in the era of emerging chemotherapy-free targeted therapies will be how to integrate alkylating agents into the treatment algorithm and whether there are still subgroups of patients with WM for whom chemoimmunotherapy is still the best choice. Data on targeted therapies, as exemplified by ibrutinib, are appealing. Notably, however, ibrutinib efficacy clearly depends on the WM genotype.[2] Intriguingly, first preliminary results suggest that chemoimmunotherapy acts independently from the genotype.[16] If this holds true, chemoimmunotherapy, including alkylating agents, would be an attractive option, particularly for patients with wildtype MYD88 and wildtype CXCR4. To that end, alkylating agents in combination with rituximab stay a powerful and cost-effective treatment option in WM currently and every new approach in WM should be judged in comparison with chemoimmunotherapy.

REFERENCES

1. Treon SP, Tripsas CK, Meid K, et al. Ibrutinib in previously treated Waldenstrom's macroglobulinemia. N Engl J Med 2015;372(15):1430–40.

2. Treon SP, Xu L, Hunter Z. MYD88 mutations and response to ibrutinib in Waldenstrom's macroglobulinemia. N Engl J Med 2015;373(6):584–6.

3. Leblond V, Kastritis E, Advani R, et al. Treatment recommendations from the Eighth International Workshop on Waldenstrom's Macroglobulinemia. Blood 2016;128(10):1321–8.

4. Buske C, Leblond V. How to manage Waldenstrom's macroglobulinemia. Leukemia 2013;27(4):762–72.
5. Tedeschi A, Benevolo G, Varettoni M, et al. Results of a phase II multicenter study of immunochemotherapy with fludarabine, cyclophosphamide and rituximab (FCR) for symptomatic waldenstrom's macroglobulinemia. Blood 2009;(114): 3692a.
6. Buske C, Hoster E, Dreyling M, et al. The addition of rituximab to front-line therapy with CHOP (R-CHOP) results in a higher response rate and longer time to treatment failure in patients with lymphoplasmacytic lymphoma: results of a randomized trial of the German Low-Grade Lymphoma Study Group (GLSG). Leukemia 2009;23(1):153–61.
7. Abonour R, Zhang L, Rajkumar V, et al. Phase II pilot study of rituximab + CHOP in patients with newly diagnosed WM, an ECOG Study (E1A02). Blood 2007;110: 3616a.
8. Dimopoulos MA, Anagnostopoulos A, Kyrtsonis MC, et al. Primary treatment of Waldenstrom macroglobulinemia with dexamethasone, rituximab, and cyclophosphamide. J Clin Oncol 2007;25(22):3344–9.
9. Dimopoulos MA, Kyrtsonis MC, Tsatalas C, et al. Primary treatment of Waldenstrom's Macroglobulinemia (WM) with dexamethasone, rituximab and cyclophosphamide. Blood 2004;104(11):752a.
10. Kastritis E, Gavriatopoulou M, Kyrtsonis MC, et al. Dexamethasone, rituximab, and cyclophosphamide as primary treatment of Waldenstrom macroglobulinemia: final analysis of a phase 2 study. Blood 2015;126(11):1392–4.
11. Rummel MJ, Niederle N, Maschmeyer G, et al. Bendamustine plus rituximab versus CHOP plus rituximab as first-line treatment for patients with indolent and mantle-cell lymphomas: an open-label, multicentre, randomised, phase 3 non-inferiority trial. Lancet 2013;381(9873):1203–10.
12. Rummel MJ, Lerchenmüller C, Greil R, et al. Bendamustin-rituximab induction followed by observation or rituximab maintenance for newly diagnosed patients with Waldenström's macroglobulinemia: results from a prospective, randomized, multicenter study (StiL NHL 7–2008 –MAINTAIN-; ClinicalTrials.gov Identifier: NCT00877214). Blood 2012;120(2739).
13. Treon SP, Hanzis C, Manning RJ, et al. Maintenance Rituximab is associated with improved clinical outcome in rituximab naive patients with Waldenstrom Macroglobulinaemia who respond to a rituximab-containing regimen. Br J Haematol 2011;154(3):357–62.
14. Marcus R, Davies A, Ando K, et al. Obinutuzumab for the first-line treatment of follicular lymphoma. N Engl J Med 2017;377(14):1331–44.
15. Herold M, Hoster E, Janssens A, et al. Immunochemotherapy with obinutuzumab or rituximab in a subset of patients in the randomised Gallium trial with previously untreated marginal zone lymphoma (MZL). Hematol Oncol 2017;35(S2):146–7.
16. Paludo J, Abeykoon JP, Shreders A, et al. Bendamustine and rituximab (BR) versus dexamethasone, rituximab, and cyclophosphamide (DRC) in patients with Waldenstrom macroglobulinemia. Ann Hematol 2018;97(8):1417–25.
17. Castillo JJ, Gustine JN, Meid K, et al. Response and survival for primary therapy combination regimens and maintenance rituximab in Waldenstrom macroglobulinaemia. Br J Haematol 2018;181(1):77–85.

Proteasome Inhibitors in Waldenström Macroglobulinemia

Efstathios Kastritis, MD*, Meletios A. Dimopoulos, MD

KEYWORDS

- Bortezomib • Carfilzomib • Oprozomib • Ixazomib • Unfolded protein response

KEY POINTS

- Proteasome inhibitors (PIs) have become an important part of WM therapy both as primary therapy and as salvage option.
- Bortezomib is the proteasome inhibitor mostly studied and with extensive clinical experience. Bortezomib is active either as a single agent and in combinations with rituximab in all disease settings.
- Bortezomib-associated neuropathy is the most common and challenging toxicity although the use of subcutaneous bortezomib and weekly regimens may reduce its frequency and severity; risk of herpes zoster reactivation is also high if no prophylaxis is given.
- Carfilzomib is a second generation PI and in combination with rituximab and dexamethasone has shown activity in WM; it has low neuropathy risk but has been associated with a potential of cardiotoxicity.
- Ixazomib is an orally available PI, has shown activity in combination with rituximab in newly diagnosed WM and a favorable toxicity profile, with low risk of neurotoxicity or cardiotoxicity. Oprozomib is another oral PI but still in earlier stages of clinical development.

INTRODUCTION

Waldenström macroglobulinemia (WM) is an incurable B-cell lymphoproliferative disorder that is characterized by the infiltration of the bone marrow by clonal lymphoplasmacytic cells and the production of monoclonal immunoglobulin M (IgM) by these cells.[1–4] WM may have a long course, even in symptomatic patients, and during the course of the disease, multiple regimens may be used to control the disease and its

Conflicts of Interest: E. Kastritis has received honoraria from Amgen, Genesis Pharma, Janssen, Takeda, and Prothena. M.A. Dimopoulos has received honoraria from Amgen, Celgene, Janssen, and Takeda.
Department of Clinical Therapeutics, National and Kapodistrian University of Athens School of Medicine, 80 Vassilisis Sofias Avenue, Athens 11528, Greece
* Corresponding author. Department of Clinical Therapeutics, National and Kapodistrian University of Athens School of Medicine, 80 Vassilisis Sofias Avenue, Athens 11528, Greece.
E-mail addresses: ekastritis@gmail.com; ekastritis@med.uoa.gr

symptoms.[2,5,6] Currently, therapy is considered only for patients with symptomatic disease, and primary options include combinations based on anti-CD20 monoclonal antibodies, mainly rituximab.[2,5,6]

In recent years, proteasome inhibitors (PIs) have become a mainstay of therapy in plasma cell malignancies but also in some specific lymphomas.[7] Regarding the treatment landscape in WM, PIs have also become part of primary and salvage options for patients with WM,[2,5,6] based on the results of several phase 2 studies, mostly with bortezomib, the first in the class of PI. In addition, new PIs have become available and may also find their way into WM therapy, such as carfilzomib, ixazomib, and oprozomib.

In this review, the authors focus on the clinical results of PI-based therapy and the challenges phased in the changing landscape of available therapies for WM.

MECHANISMS OF ACTION

PIs block degradation of ubiquitinated proteins by the proteasome, an organelle found in all cells.[8,9] Blocking proteasome activity results in the accumulation of ubiquitinated proteins and leads to dysregulation of multiple pathways within the cells but also to an increase of endoplasmatic reticulum (ER) stress. Cells that are sensitive cannot cope with the increased ER stress load, and this leads to the activation of apoptotic pathways. Although this schema may be oversimplified, cells that are most sensitive seem to be those that are producing higher amounts of protein, such as plasma cells and other B cells.[10] Different PIs have differences in their affinity for the various proteasome subunits, reversibility or nonreversibility of interaction, and pharmacokinetics. Bortezomib is the first in the class of PI and is a slowly reversible boronated inhibitor of the 26S proteasome, mostly of the chymotryptic unit of the proteasome.[11] Carfilzomib is an irreversible tetrapeptide epoxyketone–based PI (analogue of epoxomicin).[12] Ixazomib is an orally available, boronated, PI, which is metabolized to its active form,[13,14] whereas oprozomib is an oral analogue of carfilzomib.[15]

Preclinical studies have elucidated multiple mechanisms of action for PIs in WM, and bortezomib is the PI mostly studied.[16,17] Bortezomib blockade of the ubiquitin-proteasome degradation pathway affects signaling pathways that also include NF-κB,[16] which has critical function in WM cells' survival and immunoglobulin production. The induction of ER stress has also been implicated as a mechanism for bortezomib activity leading to disruption of the unfolded protein response that prompts WM cell apoptosis,[17,18] which is active in WM cell lines and in primary tumor cells. PIs may also impact the supportive bone marrow microenvironment in WM as has also been implicated for its activity in multiple myeloma.[17,18] Bortezomib has also demonstrated synergistic and/or additive preclinical activity in combination with other agents, including steroids, rituximab, and signaling inhibitors in WM cells.[19,20]

CLINICAL DATA ON THE ACTIVITY OF PROTEASOME INHIBITORS

PIs have undergone extensive clinical investigation in WM, either as a single agent or as part of combination therapies (**Table 1**). The first PI studied in the clinic was bortezomib, initially in patients with relapsed or refractory WM, and was given as a single agent and through an intravenous (IV) route.

Dimopoulos and colleagues[21] investigated the activity of single-agent bortezomib (1.3 mg/m^2 as IV push on days 1, 4, 8, and 11 of a 21-day cycle for up to 6 cycles) in 10 previously treated patients. A major response, that is, at least a partial response

Table 1
Proteasome inhibitor–based treatment studies in Waldenström macroglobulinemia

	PI/Combination	N	Disease Status	ORR, %	Major RR, %	Response Duration
Dimopoulos et al,[21] 2005	Bortezomib	10	Previously treated	80	60	>11 mo (DOR)
Treon et al,[22] 2007	Bortezomib	27	Previously treated	85	48	7 mo (TTP)
Chen et al,[23] 2007	Bortezomib	27	Untreated, previously treated	78	44	16 mo (TTP)
Leblond et al,[25] 2017	Bortezomib (± Dex after 2 cycles)	34	Previously treated	43 (after 2 cycles) 63 (after 6 cycles in N = 32)	17 (after 2 cycles) 42 (after 6 cycles in N = 32)	15.3 mo (PFS)
Ghobrial et al,[30] 2010	VR	26	Untreated	88	65	79% (1 y EFS)
Ghobrial et al,[31] 2010	VR	37	Previously treated	81	51	16 mo (TTP)
Agathocleous et al,[28] 2010	VR	10	Previously treated	90	90	N/A
Treon et al,[26] 2009; Treon et al,[27] 2015	BDR	23	Untreated	96	83	52 mo (TTP)
Dimopoulos et al,[32,33] 2013	BDR	59	Untreated	85	68	43 mo (PFS)
Ghobrial et al,[34] 2015	RVR	36	Previously treated	89	56	21 mo (PFS)
Treon et al,[39] 2014	CaRD	31	Untreated, previously treated	87	68	N/R after median follow-up of 15 mo
Vesole et al,[40] 2018	Carfilzomib/Dex	7	Previously treated	100	86	13–27 mo
Ghobrial et al,[43] 2016	Oprozomib	17	Previously treated	59	29	N/A
Castillo et al,[42] 2018	Ixazomib/Rituximab/Dex	26	Untreated	96	77	90% at 18 mo PFS

Abbreviations: DOR, duration of response; EFS, event-free survival; N/A, not available; N/R, not reached; RVR, RAD001 (Everolimus), bortezomib (Velcade), rituximab; VR, bortezomib, rituximab.

(PR), was observed in 6/10 patients (60%), whereas 2 (20%) additional patients attained a minor response for an overall response rate of 80%. The median time to a major response was 16 weeks, and the time to progression (TTP) was expected to exceed 11 months for the responders.

In a multicenter study by the Waldenström's Macroglobulinemia Clinical Trials Group, patients with previously treated WM received single-agent bortezomib (1.3 mg/m^2 IV push on days 1, 4, 8, and 11 of a 21-day cycle).[22] Twenty-seven patients received up to 8 cycles of bortezomib, and the overall and major response rates were 85% and 48%, respectively. Importantly, responses were rapid in this trial, with a median time to first and best response of 1.4 months and of 4.1 months, respectively. The median TTP for all patients was 7 months, and there was a trend for a longer median TTP in patients achieving a major response (9 months).

In a similar trial conducted by the National Cancer Institute of Canada, single-agent bortezomib was given (IV push of 1.3 mg/m^2 with the abovementioned schedule).[23] The trial enrolled 27 untreated or previously treated patients for an overall and major response rate of 78% and 44%, respectively. Again, the responses were rapid, with a median time to first response of 1.5 months, and the median progression-free survival (PFS) for all patients was 16 months. However, in this study, nodal responses were also assessed, and it was observed that these were slower than IgM responses, although occurred in most patients with a median time to response of 12 weeks. Such discordance of nodal to IgM responses has also been observed in other trials with single-agent bortezomib, including discordance between serum IgM and bone marrow burden reductions, but the clinical significance of this phenomenon is not clear.[22,24]

In a recently published prospective study from France, a different approach to bortezomib therapy was used, in which therapy started with bortezomib alone and then dexamethasone was added if the response was inadequate.[25] In this phase 2 trial, 34 patients with relapsed/refractory WM were enrolled. Bortezomib was given at 1.3 mg/m^2 IV on days 1, 4, 8, and 11 every 21 days for 6 cycles. In nonresponding patients, dexamethasone (20 mg daily for 2 days) was added to each infusion after the second cycle. Using a Bayesian statistical approach, after 2 cycles, the Bayes estimated overall response rate was 43.2 (with 95% credible interval 28.0%–59.1%) using the "informative prior". The 2-year survival rate was 84.0%, and the median PFS was 15.3 months without a difference between patients treated with or without dexamethasone. Based on this approach, the investigators concluded that dexamethasone can improve the efficacy of bortezomib and should be associated with bortezomib-based regimens.

Based on the above data, it is clear that bortezomib alone is an active agent in WM, whereas because of its mechanism of action, the available preclinical data, and also based on the extensive experience from myeloma, it is an ideal drug to combine with other WM-acting drugs. Thus, further development of bortezomib in WM followed the pathway of combinations with rituximab.

COMBINATION THERAPIES THAT INCLUDE PROTEASOME INHIBITORS
Bortezomib Combinations

To improve depth of response as well as PFS, combination therapies with bortezomib have been extensively evaluated.

The combination of bortezomib, dexamethasone, and rituximab (BDR) was investigated by the WMCTG as a primary therapy in 23 WM patients.[26] Patients received bortezomib IV at a dose of 1.3 mg/m^2 along with dexamethasone 40 mg on days 1, 4, 8, and 11, whereas rituximab was given on day 11 of each 21-day cycle. Four cycles of induction therapy were given. Twelve weeks after induction therapy completion, one cycle of therapy was given every 12 weeks for a total of 4 cycles as a maintenance therapy. The overall response rate was 96%, with 83% of patients achieving a major response. The median time to response was 1.1 months. An "IgM flare" was observed in only 9% of patients; however, those with high levels of IgM received preemptive plasmapheresis. After a long follow-up of the study, the median TTP was 52 months with this regimen.[27] However, bortezomib-related neuropathy was common and led to bortezomib discontinuation in 60% of patients, although with the longer follow-up a near complete resolution or partial resolution of treatment-related neuropathy to grade 1 was observed in most patients. Other toxicities associated with combination included dexamethasone-related hyperglycemia, myopathy, and gastritis that also prompted omission or dose reduction of steroids in many patients. Furthermore, the addition of steroids to bortezomib was deemed responsible for herpes zoster that occurred in 4 of the first 7 patients entered on this trial, and who did not receive herpes zoster prophylaxis, leading to institution of prophylaxis while on active therapy plus 6 additional months following end of therapy.

In an effort to ameliorate steroid-related toxicity and also to reduce bortezomib-associated neuropathy, Ghobrial and colleagues[30,31] and Agathocleous and colleagues[28] examined bortezomib in combination with rituximab (VR) in untreated as well as previously treated patients with WM, using a different schedule.

In the Agathocleous and colleagues[28] trial, VR was given in previously treated WM patients, in a study that also included other lymphoma histologies, and randomized between weekly and twice weekly IV bortezomib along with rituximab. Nine of 10 (90%) WM patients in this study had a major response, and 4 of these patients remained free of progression after 2 years. However, the risk of neuropathy was not impacted by treatment arm (weekly vs biweekly bortezomib administration), although only a small number of WM patients were included in each arm.

In the 2 trials led by Ghobrial and colleagues,[30,31] bortezomib was administered IV, as in the previous ones, but was given weekly at a dose of 1.6 mg/m^2 on days 1, 8, 15, every 28 days (for up to 6 cycles). Rituximab was given at the standard 375 mg/m^2 dose weekly during cycles 1 and 4, following an "extended rituximab schedule."[29] The overall response rate for the 26 untreated patients who received VR was 88%, with a major response of 65%.[30] The median TTP at the time of reporting the study was not reached, with an estimated 1-year event-free rate of 79%. Common grade 3 and 4 therapy-related adverse events included reversible neutropenia in 12%, anemia in 8%, and thrombocytopenia in 8% of patients. Regarding treatment-related neuropathy, this was observed in 15% of patients at grade 2, and in none of the patients at the grade 3 or 4 level. Among the 37 previously treated patients who received VR, the overall response rate was 81%, including 51% of patients who achieved a major response.[31] The median TTP in this study was 16.4 months. The most common grade 3 and 4 therapy-related adverse events included reversible neutropenia in 16%, anemia in 11%, and thrombocytopenia in 14%. Again, mild peripheral neuropathy (PN) grade 1 to 2 was 41% and grade ≥ 3 treatment-related PN was low and occurred in 2 patients (5%). In the above studies with VR, rituximab-related IgM flare phenomenon occurred in 20% to 30%, indicating that a different strategy should be used to ameliorate this complication by exploiting bortezomib's activity.

In a prospective, multicenter clinical trial conducted by the European Myeloma Network, a novel schedule of administration for BDR was evaluated in 59 untreated WM patients, most of which were of advanced age and with adverse prognostic factors.[32] Patients received twice weekly IV bortezomib (1.3 mg/m^2 days 1, 4, 8, and 11 of a single 21-day cycle) for the first cycle, in order to rapidly reduce IgM and avoid IgM flare when rituximab was given. Afterward, they received weekly bortezomib (at a dose of 1.6 mg/m^2 on days 1, 8, 15, and 22 of 35-day cycles) for cycles 2 to 5, along with dexamethasone (40 mg). Rituximab (at a standard dose of 375 mg/m^2) was given weekly in cycles 2 and 5. However, and unlike the WMCTG trial, no maintenance therapy was given after induction completion. An overall response rate of 85% was attained, including a major response in 68% of patients. The median PFS in this study was 43 months, and patients with very good partial response (VGPR) or better had significantly longer PFS. Treatment-related PN occurred at grade 2 in 17% and was grade 3 in 7% of patients. Importantly, rituximab-related IgM flare was observed in 11% of patients, but there was no need for plasmapheresis. An update of this study after a minimum follow-up of 6 years showed that this alkylator-free regimen was associated with a median PFS of 43 months, whereas the median duration of response for patients with at least PR was 64.5 months and the overall survival at 7 years was 66%. Importantly, no patient had developed secondary myelodysplasia, whereas transformation to high-grade lymphoma occurred in 3 patients who had received chemoimmunotherapy after BDR.[33]

The combination of the mTOR inhibitor everolimus with bortezomib and rituximab (RVR) has also been examined in a prospective trial in patients with previously treated WM.[34] Thirty-six patients received 6 cycles of RVR. Each 28-day cycle consisted of everolimus 10 mg by mouth daily, bortezomib 1.6 mg/m^2 given IV weekly on days 1, 8, 15, and for cycles 1 and 4 only, rituximab 375 mg/m^2 was given IV on days 1, 8, 15, and 22. Following 6 cycles of therapy, patients continued on everolimus alone as maintenance therapy until progression. Most patients on RVR had received prior rituximab and/or bortezomib. An overall response rate of 89%, with a major response rate of 53%, was observed in this study. The median PFS was 21 months. No grade ≥3 PN was observed in this study, although cytopenias were commonly observed that included grade ≥3 anemia (30%), neutropenia (13%), and thrombocytopenia (13%).

However, bortezomib has been clearly associated with certain toxicities, the most prominent of which is neurotoxicity.[21–23] Bortezomib-associated neuropathy is challenging to manage if unnoticeable and left without appropriate action.[35] Actually, bortezomib-related neuropathy is the most common reason for dose reductions and early discontinuation of therapy,[26,32] limiting the duration of treatment with this agent. The use of subcutaneous instead of IV bortezomib has been associated with similar efficacy and less neuropathy in patients with myeloma,[36,37] but no such direct comparisons exist in WM. Early dose adjustments, when neuropathy is still mild, and recognition of patients at risk (such as diabetics, those with prior exposure to neurotoxic drugs) are all important. Weekly versus twice-per-week dosing is also associated with lower risk of neuropathy and probably with better relative dose intensity of therapy with bortezomib. Infectious complications are not uncommon, and a risk of herpes zoster reactivation is high if no prophylaxis is given.[26] Gastrointestinal toxicity (constipation or diarrhea), conjunctivitis, and lung toxicity have also been reported with various but rather low frequencies. Generally, bortezomib has not been considered cardiotoxic, although some data may indicate some association with arrhythmias and left ventricular ejection fraction reduction.

OTHER PROTEASOME INHIBITORS
Carfilzomib

Carfilzomib is a second-generation PI, and extensive experience in myeloma patients has shown that it is associated with low neuropathy risk, although it has been associated with a potential of cardiotoxicity.[38]

WM was evaluated in combination with rituximab and dexamethasone (CaRD) in WM patients that were naive to both bortezomib and rituximab.[39] CaRD therapy consisted of IV carfilzomib given at 20 mg/m^2 (on cycle 1), and on 36 mg/m^2 thereafter (cycles 2–6), on days 1, 2 and 8, 9 with dexamethasone 20 mg on days 1, 2, 8, 9 and rituximab 375 mg/m^2 on days 2, 9 every 21 days. Maintenance therapy followed 8 weeks after cycle 6 with IV carfilzomib 36 mg/m^2 and dexamethasone 20 mg on days 1, 2 and rituximab 375 mg/m^2 on day 2 every 8 weeks for 8 cycles. The overall response rate in this study was 87%, and 68% of the patients achieved a major response. In this study, MYD88 and CXCR4 tumor mutational status were examined and did not appear to impact response attainment, although the numbers are small. With a median follow-up of 15.4 months, 20 patients remained progression-free at the time of reporting. Grade 2 PN occurred in only 1 patient with underlying disease-related PN, and no grade 3 or higher treatment-related neuropathy events were recorded. Other grade ≥ 2 toxicities included asymptomatic hyperlipasemia (41.9%), reversible neutropenia (12.9%), and cardiomyopathy in one patient (3.2%) with multiple risk factors. Declines in serum levels of IgA and IgG were common and contributed to recurring sinobronchial infections and IV immunoglobulin use in a few patients.

In a recent case series report, Vesole and colleagues[40] reported a single-center experience of carfilzomib treatment in relapsed WM treated in a phase 1b/phase 2 program. Patients received carfilzomib at 56 or 70 mg/m^2 after 20 mg/m^2 on the first 2 doses (day 1 and 2 of the first cycle), whereas dexamethasone 8 mg was administered on each day of carfilzomib therapy during the first cycle and was optional for subsequent cycles. If patients achieved less than a PR after 4 cycles, then rituximab 375 mg/m^2 was added on day 16 of each cycle, and the carfilzomib dose was decreased to 27 mg/m^2. Patients were treated to maximal response plus 2 additional cycles (for a maximum 12 cycles). Seven patients received carfilzomib, and no patient received rituximab. Among the 7 patients, 4 received carfilzomib at 70 mg/m^2 and 3 received carfilzomib at 56 mg/m^2. No dose-limiting toxicities occurred, although 6 patients reported at least 1 grade ≥ 3 adverse event and one patient discontinued treatment due to an adverse event. Two patients had neuropathy events (grade 3), whose relationship to study drug was considered probable. Six patients had a prior exposure to bortezomib, and 2 were refractory. All patients achieved a minor response (MR) or better, including 1 stringent complete response (sCR) (overall 1 sCR, 3 PRs, 2 VGPRs, and 1 MR). The 2 patients that were bortezomib refractory achieved a PR. In this small series of patients, 6/7 patients did not have a PD at a follow-up time of 13 to 27 months.

Oral Proteasome Inhibitors

Ixazomib is an oral boronated PI that has now been approved for use in patients with myeloma in combination with lenalidomide and dexamethasone,[41] whereas an extensive clinical program is running and several clinical studies recruit patients in different clinical settings.

Castillo and colleagues[42] recently presented the results of a prospective phase 2 study in which oral ixazomib was given in combination with dexamethasone and rituximab (IDR) in 26 symptomatic, previously untreated patients with WM. Ixazomib was given at 4 mg with dexamethasone at 20 mg, on days 1, 8, and 15 every 28 days for induction cycles 1 and 2 (as an induction), and then in combination with rituximab 375 mg/m^2 IV, on day 1 of cycles 3 to 6. Maintenance therapy followed 8 weeks later with IDR given every 8 weeks for 6 cycles. All patients were evaluated for MYD88 and CXCR4 mutational status and were MYD88 L265P mutated, whereas 15 patients

(58%) had a CXCR4 mutation. The median time to response was 8 weeks, which was longer however (at 12 weeks) in WM patients with CXCR4 mutations (log-rank $P = .03$). The overall response rate was 96% (including VGPR 15%, PR 62%, MR 19%) with a major response rate (VGPR + PR) of 77%, but it was not impacted by CXCR4 mutations. With a median follow-up of 18 months, the median PFS was not reached, and the 18-month PFS rate was 90% (95% confidence interval 65%– 97%). Grade $\geq$2 adverse events included infusion-related reactions (19%), rash (8%), and insomnia (8%). However, ixazomib was not associated with clinically significant risk of neuropathy.

Oprozomib is an oral epoxyketone proteasome inhibitor that is an analogue of carfilzomib. The clinical development of oprozomib has been delayed because of gastrointestinal toxicity issues. The schedule of administration of oprozomib has not been fully optimized, and 2 different schedules have been evaluated in phase 1 and 2 studies. Two schedules of oprozomib given once daily either on days 1 to 5 (5/14 schedule) or on days 1, 2, 8, and 9 (2/7 schedule) of a 14-day treatment cycle have been evaluated. An overall response rate of 59% with a major response rate of 29% was observed in a phase 2 study in 17 previously treated WM patients treated with single-agent oprozomib.[43] However, gastrointestinal intolerance was prominent with oprozomib necessitating intensive antiemetic use. Although the activity of the drug seems to be high, it is still very early for oprozomib to be placed in the armamentarium of available PIs for WM.

WHERE DO PROTEASOME INHIBITORS FIT IN THE CURRENT TREATMENT RECOMMENDATIONS?

PIs have prominent activity in WM, in all disease settings, either as single agents or in combinations with other active drugs. The major advantages of PIs are that they are fast acting, reduce IgM levels quite rapidly, are non-myelotoxic, are not associated with a risk of secondary malignancies or myelodysplasia, and can be easily combined because they have nonoverlapping toxicities with most other commonly used drugs. The effect of MYD88 and CXCR4 mutational status on PI activity is unclear and less prominent than on ibrutinib efficacy. Bortezomib is the main PIs for which there is a significant amount of data and long-term experience, whereas carfilzomib use has less published data. At the moment, a randomized phase 3 study evaluates the role of addition of bortezomib to standard DRC regimen (dexamethasone, rituximab, and cyclophosphamide) in previously untreated symptomatic patients with WM (NCT01788020). The results of this study will elucidate the role of adding a PI at the frontline over a standard effective WM regimen. Ixazomib is the first oral PI that has been approved for use in myeloma patients. Also, there are data from a phase 2 study in newly diagnosed WM, whereas another ongoing phase 2 study evaluates ixazomib-rituximab combination in relapsed or refractory WM. The toxicities of PIs are different with bortezomib being associated mainly with neurotoxicity, carfilzomib with a risk of cardiotoxicity, whereas ixazomib is less neurotoxic but may have some gastrointestinal toxicity.

Bortezomib-containing combinations can be considered an option for the primary therapy for patients with high levels and in need for rapid reduction of IgM, such as those with symptomatic hyperviscosity or at risk for clinically significant IgM flare.[5] Bortezomib induction followed by bortezomib-rituximab has been used to avoid IgM flare.[32] When myelotoxicity is undesirable, bortezomib with rituximab may also be a primary option.[2,5,6,44] Carfilzomib is not widely available for WM but could be considered a neuropathy-sparing PI. Ixazomib may also be a good alternative if a PI is needed, but still data are limited and are not available for WM outside clinical trials.

However, the major change in the therapy for MW has been the introduction of ibrutinib and other BTK inhibitors.[45,46] Ibrutinib has shown substantial activity and is recommended at least for patients who relapse or have refractory disease, especially those with rituximab-refractory disease.[5,44] There are still limited data on the management and outcomes of those patients failing ibrutinib, but it seems that PIs could be a good option for patients who fail ibrutinib therapy, as shown by a recent report of patients who failed or discontinued ibrutinib due to toxicity.[47]

In summary, PIs have shown significant activity in WM; the high rates of efficacy, particularly in combination therapy, as well as their overall tolerability, have resulted in their adoption as important mainstays of WM therapy. The development of strategies to mitigate neuropathy risk of PIs, including use of weekly subcutaneous administration for bortezomib and exploration of novel neuropathy-sparing agents such carfilzomib and ixazomib will invariably lead to further advances in the use of this class of agents in the treatment of WM. Even in the era of BTK inhibitors, PIs will remain a major option for newly diagnosed and relapsed or refractory WM patients.

REFERENCES

1. Treon SP, Dimopoulos M, Kyle RA. Defining Waldenstrom's macroglobulinemia. Semin Oncol 2003;30(2):107–9.
2. Kapoor P, Ansell SM, Fonseca R, et al. Diagnosis and management of Waldenstrom macroglobulinemia: mayo stratification of macroglobulinemia and risk-adapted therapy (mSMART) guidelines 2016. JAMA Oncol 2017;3(9): 1257–65.
3. Dimopoulos MA, Panayiotidis P, Moulopoulos LA, et al. Waldenstrom's macroglobulinemia: clinical features, complications, and management. J Clin Oncol 2000;18(1):214–26.
4. Owen RG, Treon SP, Al-Katib A, et al. Clinicopathological definition of Waldenstrom's macroglobulinemia: consensus panel recommendations from the Second International Workshop on Waldenstrom's macroglobulinemia. Semin Oncol 2003; 30(2):110–5.
5. Leblond V, Kastritis E, Advani R, et al. Treatment recommendations from the Eighth International Workshop on Waldenstrom's macroglobulinemia. Blood 2016;128(10):1321–8.
6. Dimopoulos MA, Kastritis E, Owen RG, et al. Treatment recommendations for patients with Waldenstrom macroglobulinemia (WM) and related disorders: IWWM-7 consensus. Blood 2014;124(9):1404–11.
7. Gandolfi S, Laubach JP, Hideshima T, et al. The proteasome and proteasome inhibitors in multiple myeloma. Cancer Metastasis Rev 2017;36(4):561–84.
8. Lee AH, Iwakoshi NN, Anderson KC, et al. Proteasome inhibitors disrupt the unfolded protein response in myeloma cells. Proc Natl Acad Sci U S A 2003; 100(17):9946–51.
9. Mitsiades CS, Mitsiades N, Hideshima T, et al. Proteasome inhibition as a therapeutic strategy for hematologic malignancies. Expert Rev Anticancer Ther 2005; 5(3):465–76.
10. Meister S, Schubert U, Neubert K, et al. Extensive immunoglobulin production sensitizes myeloma cells for proteasome inhibition. Cancer Res 2007;67(4): 1783–92.
11. Mitsiades N, Mitsiades CS, Richardson PG, et al. The proteasome inhibitor PS-341 potentiates sensitivity of multiple myeloma cells to conventional chemotherapeutic agents: therapeutic applications. Blood 2003;101(6):2377–80.

12. Kuhn DJ, Chen Q, Voorhees PM, et al. Potent activity of carfilzomib, a novel, irreversible inhibitor of the ubiquitin-proteasome pathway, against preclinical models of multiple myeloma. Blood 2007;110(9):3281–90.

13. Chauhan D, Tian Z, Zhou B, et al. In vitro and in vivo selective antitumor activity of a novel orally bioavailable proteasome inhibitor MLN9708 against multiple myeloma cells. Clin Cancer Res 2011;17(16):5311–21.

14. Kupperman E, Lee EC, Cao Y, et al. Evaluation of the proteasome inhibitor MLN9708 in preclinical models of human cancer. Cancer Res 2010;70(5): 1970–80.

15. Hurchla MA, Garcia-Gomez A, Hornick MC, et al. The epoxyketone-based proteasome inhibitors carfilzomib and orally bioavailable oprozomib have anti-resorptive and bone-anabolic activity in addition to anti-myeloma effects. Leukemia 2013; 27(2):430–40.

16. Leleu X, Eeckhoute J, Jia X, et al. Targeting NF-kappaB in Waldenstrom macroglobulinemia. Blood 2008;111(10):5068–77.

17. Roccaro AM, Leleu X, Sacco A, et al. Dual targeting of the proteasome regulates survival and homing in Waldenstrom macroglobulinemia. Blood 2008;111(9): 4752–63.

18. Sacco A, Aujay M, Morgan B, et al. Carfilzomib-dependent selective inhibition of the chymotrypsin-like activity of the proteasome leads to antitumor activity in Waldenstrom's macroglobulinemia. Clin Cancer Res 2011;17(7):1753–64.

19. Wang M, Han XH, Zhang L, et al. Bortezomib is synergistic with rituximab and cyclophosphamide in inducing apoptosis of mantle cell lymphoma cells in vitro and in vivo. Leukemia 2008;22(1):179–85.

20. Alinari L, White VL, Earl CT, et al. Combination bortezomib and rituximab treatment affects multiple survival and death pathways to promote apoptosis in mantle cell lymphoma. MAbs 2009;1(1):31–40.

21. Dimopoulos MA, Anagnostopoulos A, Kyrtsonis MC, et al. Treatment of relapsed or refractory Waldenstrom's macroglobulinemia with bortezomib. Haematologica 2005;90(12):1655–8.

22. Treon SP, Hunter ZR, Matous J, et al. Multicenter clinical trial of bortezomib in relapsed/refractory Waldenstrom's macroglobulinemia: results of WMCTG trial 03-248. Clin Cancer Res 2007;13(11):3320–5.

23. Chen CI, Kouroukis CT, White D, et al. Bortezomib is active in patients with untreated or relapsed Waldenstrom's macroglobulinemia: a phase II study of the National Cancer Institute of Canada Clinical Trials Group. J Clin Oncol 2007; 25(12):1570–5.

24. Strauss SJ, Maharaj L, Hoare S, et al. Bortezomib therapy in patients with relapsed or refractory lymphoma: potential correlation of in vitro sensitivity and tumor necrosis factor alpha response with clinical activity. J Clin Oncol 2006; 24(13):2105–12.

25. Leblond V, Morel P, Dilhuidy MS, et al. A phase II Bayesian sequential clinical trial in advanced Waldenstrom macroglobulinemia patients treated with bortezomib: interest of addition of dexamethasone. Leuk Lymphoma 2017;58(11):2615–23.

26. Treon SP, Ioakimidis L, Soumerai JD, et al. Primary therapy of Waldenstrom macroglobulinemia with bortezomib, dexamethasone, and rituximab: WMCTG clinical trial 05-180. J Clin Oncol 2009;27(23):3830–5.

27. Treon SP, Meid K, Gustine J, et al. Long-term outcome of a prospective study of bortezomib, dexamethasone and rituximab (BDR) in previously untreated, symptomatic patients with Waldenstrom's macroglobulinemia. Blood 2015;126(23): 1833.

28. Agathocleous A, Rohatiner A, Rule S, et al. Weekly versus twice weekly bortezomib given in conjunction with rituximab, in patients with recurrent follicular lymphoma, mantle cell lymphoma and Waldenstrom macroglobulinaemia. Br J Haematol 2010;151(4):346–53.

29. Dimopoulos MA, Zervas C, Zomas A, et al. Extended rituximab therapy for previously untreated patients with Waldenstrom's macroglobulinemia. Clin Lymphoma 2002;3(3):163–6.

30. Ghobrial IM, Xie W, Padmanabhan S, et al. Phase II trial of weekly bortezomib in combination with rituximab in untreated patients with Waldenstrom Macroglobulinemia. Am J Hematol 2010;85(9):670–4.

31. Ghobrial IM, Hong F, Padmanabhan S, et al. Phase II trial of weekly bortezomib in combination with rituximab in relapsed or relapsed and refractory Waldenstrom macroglobulinemia. J Clin Oncol 2010;28(8):1422–8.

32. Dimopoulos MA, Garcia-Sanz R, Gavriatopoulou M, et al. Primary therapy of Waldenstrom macroglobulinemia (WM) with weekly bortezomib, low-dose dexamethasone, and rituximab (BDR): long-term results of a phase 2 study of the European Myeloma Network (EMN). Blood 2013;122(19):3276–82.

33. Gavriatopoulou M, Garcia-Sanz R, Kastritis E, et al. BDR in newly diagnosed patients with WM: final analysis of a phase 2 study after a minimum follow-up of 6 years. Blood 2017;129(4):456–9.

34. Ghobrial IM, Redd R, Armand P, et al. Phase I/II trial of everolimus in combination with bortezomib and rituximab (RVR) in relapsed/refractory Waldenstrom macroglobulinemia. Leukemia 2015;29(12):2338–46.

35. Arastu-Kapur S, Anderl JL, Kraus M, et al. Nonproteasomal targets of the proteasome inhibitors bortezomib and carfilzomib: a link to clinical adverse events. Clin Cancer Res 2011;17(9):2734–43.

36. Moreau P, Pylypenko H, Grosicki S, et al. Subcutaneous versus intravenous administration of bortezomib in patients with relapsed multiple myeloma: a randomised, phase 3, non-inferiority study. Lancet Oncol 2011;12(5):431–40.

37. Moreau P, Coiteux V, Hulin C, et al. Prospective comparison of subcutaneous versus intravenous administration of bortezomib in patients with multiple myeloma. Haematologica 2008;93(12):1908–11.

38. Dimopoulos MA, Roussou M, Gavriatopoulou M, et al. Cardiac and renal complications of carfilzomib in patients with multiple myeloma. Blood Adv 2017;1(7):449–54.

39. Treon SP, Tripsas CK, Meid K, et al. Carfilzomib, rituximab, and dexamethasone (CaRD) treatment offers a neuropathy-sparing approach for treating Waldenstrom's macroglobulinemia. Blood 2014;124(4):503–10.

40. Vesole DH, Richter J, Biran N, et al. Carfilzomib as salvage therapy in Waldenstrom macroglobulinemia: a case series. Leuk Lymphoma 2018;59(1):259–61.

41. Moreau P, Masszi T, Grzasko N, et al. Oral ixazomib, lenalidomide, and dexamethasone for multiple myeloma. N Engl J Med 2016;374(17):1621–34.

42. Castillo JJ, Meid K, Gustine J, et al. Prospective clinical trial of ixazomib, dexamethasone and rituximab as primary therapy in Waldenström macroglobulinemia. Clin Cancer Res 2018. Epub ahead of print.

43. Ghobrial IM, Savona MR, Vij R, et al. Final results from a multicenter, open-label, dose-escalation phase 1b/2 study of single-agent oprozomib in patients with hematologic malignancies. Blood 2016;128(22):2110.

44. Kastritis E, Dimopoulos MA. Current therapy guidelines for Waldenstrom's macroglobulinaemia. Best Pract Res Clin Haematol 2016;29(2):194–205.

45. Treon SP, Tripsas CK, Meid K, et al. Ibrutinib in previously treated Waldenstrom's macroglobulinemia. N Engl J Med 2015;372(15):1430–40.
46. Dimopoulos MA, Trotman J, Tedeschi A, et al. Ibrutinib for patients with rituximab-refractory Waldenstrom's macroglobulinaemia (iNNOVATE): an open-label sub-study of an international, multicentre, phase 3 trial. Lancet Oncol 2017;18(2): 241–50.
47. Gustine J, Meid K, Dubeau T, et al. Ibrutinib discontinuation in Waldenström macroglobulinemia: etiologies, outcomes, and IgM rebound. Blood 2017; 130(Suppl 1):802.

Monoclonal Antibodies for Waldenström Macroglobulinemia

Andres Dominguez, MD[a], Efstathios Kastritis, MD[b],
Jorge J. Castillo, MD[c],*

KEYWORDS

- Mechanism of action • Treatment • Monoclonal antibodies
- Waldenström macroglobulinemia

KEY POINTS

- For the last 2 decades, anti-CD20 monoclonal antibodies have revolutionized the treatment of patients with B-cell lymphomas. These agents have shown efficacy when used as single agents and also have improved response and survival rates when added to chemotherapy.
- Monoclonal antibodies are safe and effective as well in patients with Waldenström macroglobulinemia (WM).
- The purpose of the present article is to briefly review the mechanism of action of monoclonal antibodies and to discuss current clinical data supporting their use in patients with WM.
- This review focuses on retrospective as well as clinical trials on the anti-CD20 antibodies rituximab, ofatumumab, and obinutuzumab, the anti-CD38 antibody daratumumab, and the anti-CXCR4 antibody ulocuplumab.

INTRODUCTION

The anti-CD20 monoclonal antibody rituximab is inarguably the most commonly used agent in patients with Waldenström macroglobulinemia (WM). In addition to its efficacy, the favorable toxicity profile of rituximab has allowed a broad use in WM. Rituximab is used alone or in combination with chemotherapy, such as cyclophosphamide and bendamustine, and proteasome inhibitors, such as bortezomib and carfilzomib.

New monoclonal antibodies have also been shown to be safe and effective in patients with WM, including the anti-CD20 monoclonal antibody ofatumumab, while

[a] Department of Internal Medicine, Fundación Valle del Lili, CES University, Cali, Colombia;
[b] Department of Clinical Therapeutics, National and Kapodistrian University, Athens, Greece;
[c] Bing Center for Waldenstrom Macroglobulinemia, Dana-Farber Cancer Institute, Harvard Medical School, 450 Brookline Avenue, Mayer 221, Boston, MA 02215, USA
* Corresponding author.
E-mail address: jorgej_castillo@dfci.harvard.edu

Hematol Oncol Clin N Am 32 (2018) 841–852
https://doi.org/10.1016/j.hoc.2018.05.010
0889-8588/18/© 2018 Elsevier Inc. All rights reserved.

hemonc.theclinics.com

obinutuzumab is currently being evaluated in clinical trials. Other targets for monoclonal antibody therapy include surface antigen CD38, of great success in patients with myeloma, and CXCR4, which is of interest given the presence of CXCR4 mutations in approximately 40% of patients with WM.

In this article, the authors review the mechanism of action of monoclonal antibodies, the available data supporting the use of these agents in WM, as well as ongoing clinical trials.

MECHANISMS OF ACTION OF MONOCLONAL ANTIBODIES

The fundamental basis of antibody-based therapy dates back to the original observations of antigen expression by tumor cells through serologic techniques in the 1960s. The definition of cell surface antigens that are expressed by human cancers has revealed a broad array of targets that are overexpressed, mutated, or selectively expressed compared with normal tissues.[1]

Monoclonal antibodies have a fixed effector cell binding (Fc) region and a variable region with affinity toward a specific antigen. Antibodies can mediate cytotoxicity toward tumor cells via both direct and indirect mechanisms based on the target. Direct cytotoxicity of tumor cells can occur through transmembrane signaling, and recruitment of effector cells (ie, natural killer [NK] cells, macrophages, neutrophils) that mediate antibody-dependent cell cytotoxicity and phagocytosis (ADCC and ADCP, respectively), and complement that mediates complement-dependent cytotoxicity (CDC). Indirect cytotoxicity can occur by interfering with both the interaction of a tumor cell with the microenvironment-generated survival signal and its binding to soluble factors that enhance tumor cell survival.[2]

ADCC, ADCP, and CDC are promoted when the variable region of the monoclonal antibody binds to its specific antigen, and the Fc region of the monoclonal antibody interacts with the Fc receptor of an effector cell (eg, NK cell or cytotoxic T cells) or macrophage.[3] Fc receptor crosslinking activates effector cells and mediates the release of enzymes and peptides, by the effector cell, that mediates target cell killing. Through a similar mechanism, Fc receptor crosslinking also activates monocytes and macrophages promoting ADCP.[4] The Fc portion of the monoclonal antibody may interact with C1q and initiate the classical pathway of complement activation, specifically through C3b and subsequent formation of the membrane attack complex, inducing cell killing through osmotic stress.[5] C3b also acts as an opsonizing molecule further inducing ADCC and ADCP. Most of tumor cells have an overexpression of growth receptors that give them intracellular signals for proliferation and survival. Monoclonal antibodies can diminish signaling through modulation of membrane-bound receptors, which in turn slows the rates of growth, activates intracellular apoptosis pathways, and/or sensitizes cells to cytotoxic agents.[2]

RITUXIMAB

Rituximab is a chimeric murine/human monoclonal antibody directed against the surface antigen CD20, which is expressed selectively on B-cells from the pre-B-cell stage until postgerminal center cells that differentiate to become plasma cells.[2] CD20 seems to be an excellent target for antibody-based therapy in mature B-cell malignancies, unlike other antigens, because it is not shed or internalized in resting normal B cells.[6] As with other immunoglobulin G1 (IgG1) antibodies used in clinical practice, rituximab mediates it effects by CDC, ADCC, and direct apoptosis. Rituximab was the first approved therapeutic monoclonal antibody for the treatment of cancer. CD20 is a suitable target for therapy in WM as most malignant lymphoplasmacytic cells avidly express CD20 on the membrane.[7]

Despite being the most commonly used agent for WM in the United States,[8] rituximab has not been formally approved for the treatment of WM. Rituximab has been approved by the US Food and Drug Administration (FDA) for the treatment of patients with non-Hodgkin lymphoma (NHL), and it can be used alone or in combination for the following:

- Relapsed or refractory, low-grade or follicular, CD20-positive B-cell NHL as a single agent
- Previously untreated follicular, CD20-positive, B-cell NHL in combination with first-line chemotherapy and, in patients achieving a complete or PR to Rituximab in combination with chemotherapy, as single-agent maintenance therapy
- Nonprogressing (including stable disease), low-grade, CD20-positive, B-cell NHL as a single agent after first-line cyclophosphamide, vincristine, and prednisone chemotherapy
- Previously untreated diffuse large B-cell, CD20-positive NHL in combination with cyclophosphamide, doxorubicin, vincristine, and prednisone (CHOP) or other anthracycline-based chemotherapy regimens

Single-Agent Rituximab

Byrd and colleagues[9] first reported a small retrospective series of patients with resistant WM who were treated with single-agent rituximab and showed that 3 of 7 patients achieved a partial response (PR).[9] Treon and colleagues[10] published a large retrospective series of 30 patients with WM who were treated with single-agent rituximab. Eight (27%) and 10 (33%) patients achieved PR and minor response (mR), respectively, and 9 (30%) patients demonstrated stable disease. Moreover, 63% and 50% of patients had improvements in hematocrit and platelet counts, respectively.

Dimopoulos and colleagues[11] reported on a prospective, nonrandomized phase 2 study that included 27 patients with WM that evaluated the activity of rituximab in previously untreated (n = 15) and pretreated (n = 12) patients. Rituximab was administered at a dose of 375 mg/m^2 intravenous (IV) weekly for 4 consecutive weeks, and 3 months after completion of rituximab, patients with no evidence of progression received another 4 weekly doses of rituximab. Twelve (44%) patients achieved a PR with a median time to response (TTR) of 3.3 months. All adverse events were grade 1 or 2, and most of them were infusion reactions readily reversible after reducing the infusion rate. In an updated report on 17 previously untreated patients, using an extended treatment approach in those patients without evidence of progressive disease at 3 months, 35% achieved a PR after extended treatment with rituximab.[12] For all patients, the median TTR was 3 months, and the median time to progression (TTP) was 13 months. Treon and colleagues[13] also published a nonrandomized phase 2 trial with an extended dose schedule of rituximab. Of 26 patients who completed intended therapy, 14 (48%) achieved a PR and 5 (17%) achieved an mR. There was a difference in the rate of response between patients with different levels of IgM. The major response rate in WM patients with serum IgM level less than 6000 mg/dL was 75%, compared with only 20% in patients with serum IgM level greater than 6000 mg/dL. The median time to best response was 17 months, with patients continuing to show reduction in IgM several months after rituximab completion.

In a multicenter phase 2 study (ECOG 3A98) designed to evaluate the clinical response in patients with untreated and treated WM, 69 patients, 34 untreated and 35 previously treated, were included.[14] Overall, 52% achieved a response

(28% PR and 25% mR), with no detectable differences between previously treated and untreated patients. The median response duration for untreated patients was 27 months, and 40% of the patients experienced grade 3 adverse events, mainly infusion reactions.

Of note, a transient increase in serum IgM levels is observed in about 50% of patients who received rituximab as monotherapy, also known as "IgM flare."[15,16] IgM flare occurs mostly at the beginning of treatment; 73% of the patients presented a >25% elevation in the IgM levels at 12 weeks. This phenomenon, however, is not associated with a higher risk of treatment failure, but the IgM flare can lead to hyperviscosity-related complications, especially in patients with serum IgM level greater than 4000 mg/dL in whom initial therapy with rituximab should be undertaken with caution and appropriate monitoring.[17] The risk of IgM flare might be lower when rituximab is administered in combination with chemotherapy and especially with proteasome inhibitors.

Rituximab-Containing Combinations

As shown above, rituximab as monotherapy is effective with overall response rate (ORR) between 30% and 50%, and given its relatively benign toxicity profile, rituximab is a great candidate for combination with other agents. As summarized in **Table 1**, there are numerous retrospective and prospective studies that have evaluated rituximab in combination with alkylating agents (eg, bendamustine and cyclophosphamide), purine analogues (eg, fludarabine), and proteasome inhibitors (eg, bortezomib and carfilzomib). These combinations have demonstrated an improvement in response rates, with ORR between 80% and 90% and major response rates between 60% and 80%. Progression-free survival (PFS) rates have also improved with the addition of rituximab to chemotherapy and proteasome inhibitors. Rituximab has also been combined with immunomodulating drugs, such as thalidomide and

Table 1
Selected prospective studies evaluating rituximab-containing combination regimens in patients with Waldenström macroglobulinemia

Combination	N	Treatment Naive, %	Overall Response, %	Major Response, %	Median PFS, mo
Rituximab + Cyclophosphamide + Dexamethasone[48]	72	100	83	75	35
Rituximab + CHOP[49]	23	100	92	NA	63
Rituximab + Fludarabine[50]	43	63	95	86	51
Rituximab + Fludarabine + Cyclophosphamide[51]	43	65	79	74	50
Rituximab + Bendamustine[52]	21	100	95	NA	69
Rituximab + Bortezomib + Dexamethasone[53]	23	100	96	83	66
Rituximab + Bortezomib + Dexamethasone[54]	59	100	85	68	43
Rituximab + Carfilzomib + Dexamethasone[55]	31	90	87	68	46
Rituximab + Dexamethasone + Ixazomib[56]	26	100	96	77	Not reached at 22 mo

Abbreviation: NA, not available.

lenalidomide, with lower rates of success and higher rates of toxicity than with other combinations.[18,19]

MAINTENANCE RITUXIMAB

The use of rituximab as maintenance therapy in patients who have accomplished at least an mR to rituximab-containing induction regimens has become increasingly common in the last 10 years. Reports between 2002 and 2010 of improved categorical responses, better PFS, and better overall survival (OS) with maintenance therapy in other indolent lymphoma subtypes have prompted the study of this strategy in WM patients.

Treon and colleagues[20] examined the outcome of 248 WM patients (70% previously untreated) who responded to rituximab-containing induction regimens and subsequently received (n = 86; 35%) or did not receive (n = 162; 65%) rituximab as maintenance therapy. Categorical responses upgraded in 42% of patients who received rituximab maintenance, whereas responses upgraded in 10% of patients who did not receive maintenance. Both median PFS (56 vs 28 months, respectively) and median OS (not reached vs 116 months, respectively) were longer in patients who received rituximab maintenance than in patients who did not. An increase in the rate of infections, especially sinopulmonary infections, was observed in patients who received rituximab maintenance.

In another retrospective study, Castillo and colleagues[21] analyzed the role of maintenance therapy with rituximab in previously untreated patients who had just completed induction therapy with Benda-R (bendamustine-rituximab), BDR (bortezomib-dexamethasone-rituximab), or CDR (cyclophosphamide-dexamethasone-rituximab). Rituximab maintenance therapy was administered as a 375 mg/m^2 IV infusion every 2 to 3 months for up to 2 years. Of the 182 patients included in the study (31% received frontline therapy with Benda-R, 48% received BDR, and 21% received CDR), 116 (64%) received maintenance therapy with rituximab. Maintenance rituximab was associated with a better PFS and OS, when analyzed as a time-varying covariate in multivariate models. In these models, the risk of death and/or progression was 46% lower in patients who received maintenance rituximab. The median PFS in patients who received maintenance rituximab was 6.8 years versus 2.8 years in patients who did not. The 5- and 10-year overall survival rates for patients who received maintenance rituximab were 95% and 84%, respectively, compared with 84% and 66% in patients who did not receive maintenance therapy, for a decrease in the risk of dying of any cause of 28% associated with maintenance rituximab.

These results from retrospective studies indicate that some patients may benefit from maintenance therapy, but prospective data are still lacking. A prospective study (MAINTAIN) evaluating the role of maintenance rituximab after Benda-R in patients with indolent lymphomas, including WM, is currently ongoing in Germany, and the results are eagerly awaited (NCT00877214).

OFATUMUMAB

Ofatumumab is a fully human anti-CD20 monoclonal antibody that binds to a different epitope than rituximab.[22] This epitope is located on the smaller extracellular loop of CD20 with a reduced off rate, allowing for slower release from the target. In preclinical studies, ofatumumab induced cell killing when incubated with plasma alone, confirming its role as a potent CDC inducer. In this study, ofatumumab exhibited cell killing activity against low CD20-expressing, rituximab-resistant chronic lymphocytic leukemia (CLL) cells.[23] Another study showed that ofatumumab induced cell lysis at lower

CD20 concentrations (~4500 molecules), when compared with rituximab, which required at least 30,000 molecules to elicit activity. Ofatumumab was also shown to have a more rapid onset of cellular changes associated with apoptosis than rituximab at 114 versus 418 seconds, respectively. Finally, ofatumumab showed activity against cell lines with high levels of CD55 and CD59. These molecules inactivate complement, and high levels of CD55 and CD59 might be associated with rituximab resistance.[24]

Ofatumumab is currently approved by the FDA for patients with CLL:

- In combination with chlorambucil, for the treatment of previously untreated patients with CLL for whom fludarabine-based therapy is considered inappropriate
- In combination with fludarabine and cyclophosphamide for the treatment of patients with relapsed CLL
- For extended treatment of patients who are in complete response or PR after at least 2 lines of therapy for recurrent or progressive CLL
- For the treatment of patients with CLL refractory to fludarabine and alemtuzumab

The activity of ofatumumab in WM has been evaluated in both prospective and retrospective studies. A prospective phase 2 study evaluated ofatumumab as a single agent in 37 patients with WM,[25] which were divided into 2 treatment groups. Group A (n = 15) received ofatumumab 300 mg IV on week 1 followed by 1000 mg IV once weekly for 3 weeks. Group B (n = 22) received ofatumumab 300 mg IV on week 1 followed by 2000 mg IV once weekly for 4 weeks. Patients with stable disease or with an mR at 16 weeks could receive a redosing cycle of ofatumumab 300 mg IV on week 1 followed by 2000 mg IV once weekly for 4 weeks. A third of the patients (n = 13) received ofatumumab redosing. The median age was 63 years; the median serum IgM and hemoglobin levels were 3110 mg/dL and 9.8 g/dL, respectively. A quarter of the patients (24%) were previously untreated and had received a median of 3 prior therapies. Most previously treated patients (89%) had been exposed to rituximab. The median ORR after cycle 1 was 51% (PR 32%, mR 19%) and after redosing was 59% (PR 41%, mR 19%). Better ORR was seen in previously untreated patients (67% vs 57%), without previous exposure to rituximab (75% vs 52%), and in patients with baseline serum IgM less than 4000 mg/dL (64% vs 50%). The median TTR was 2.6 months, and the median PFS for all patients was 18 months. There were no differences in TTR of PFS between groups. The most frequent adverse events were urticaria (35%), pruritus (35%), throat irritation (27%), and flushing (27%). The most common grade 3 or 4 adverse events were infusion reaction (11%), chest pain (5%), hemolysis (5%), and neutropenia (5%). Two patients, both on group B, experienced an IgM flare, with increases in serum IgM of 79% and 240%, peaking at day 42 and 37, and achieving a response at day 356 and 93, respectively.

The combination of fludarabine, cyclophosphamide, and ofatumumab was evaluated in 12 patients with relapsed/refractory WM.[26] The study enrollment goal was 30 patients, but it was terminated earlier because of low accrual rate. Fludarabine 25 mg/m^2 and cyclophosphamide 250 mg/m^2 were given IV for 3 consecutive days every 28 days for 4 cycles. Ofatumumab 300 mg IV was given on day 1 followed by 1000 mg IV on day 8 of cycle 1, and then 1000 mg IV on day 1 of cycles 2 to 4. The median age was 69 years, and 50% of the patients were men. The median serum IgM levels were 4700 mg/dL. Patients had received a median of 1 prior therapy. All patients had received rituximab, and 25% were rituximab refractory. The ORR was 92% (Very Good Partial Response 17%, PR 67%, mR 8%). The median TTR was 2.2 months, and the 2-year PFS was 80%. Grade 3 or 4 neutropenia occurred in 92% of patients, and 1 patient had neutropenic fever. A grade 2 infusion reaction occurred in 1 patient with a history of rituximab intolerance. No IgM flare was observed. There is limited experience with the combination of bendamustine and ofatumumab in patients with relapsed and/or refractory WM, and the combination appears to be safe and effective.[27]

The National Comprehensive Cancer Network considers the use of ofatumumab useful in certain circumstances, especially in patients who are intolerant to rituximab. In these patients, ofatumumab can be used as a single agent or in combination with other agents as a replacement to rituximab. Ofatumumab intolerance has been reported in 20% of patients who are intolerant to rituximab.[28]

A prospective phase 2 study evaluating the combination of bortezomib and ofatumumab as primary therapy in patients with WM was terminated early, after enrolling only 3 participants, because of withdrawal of funding (NCT01536067).

OBINUTUZUMAB

Obinutuzumab is a type II, humanized anti-CD20 monoclonal antibody, which was glycoengineered to prevent the addition of a fucose sugar residue to IgG oligosaccharides in the Fc region of the molecule. Such modifications, in addition to binding to a unique epitope in CD20, enhance the binding affinity to the FcγRIII on immune effector cells.[29] In contrast to type I anti-CD20 antibodies, binding of type II antibodies to CD20 does not lead to internalization of CD20 in lipid rafts. These features enhance direct cell death, ADCC, and ADCP, and decrease CDC. Preclinically, obinutuzumab has been shown to elicit direct cell death at faster rates than rituximab and ofatumumab, due at least in part to the production of reactive oxygen species.[30,31] Although obinutuzumab has comparable ADCP, it seems to induce stronger ADCC than rituximab and ofatumumab, by more efficiently recruiting additional NK cells.[30–32] In vivo, obinutuzumab induced complete tumor regression in human lymphoma xenograft models at doses of 30 mg/kg, whereas rituximab and ofatumumab did not induce tumor regression at equivalent doses.[33]

Obinutuzumab is approved by the FDA for patients with CLL and follicular lymphoma (FL):

- In combination with chlorambucil, for the treatment of patients with previously untreated CLL.
- In combination with bendamustine followed by obinutuzumab monotherapy, for the treatment of patients with FL who relapsed after, or are refractory to, a rituximab-containing regimen.
- In combination with chemotherapy followed by obinutuzumab monotherapy in patients achieving at least a partial remission, for the treatment of adult patients with previously untreated stage II bulky, III, or IV FL.

A prospective phase 2 study evaluating idelalisib in combination with obinutuzumab in WM is ongoing (RemodelWM3; NCT02962401). The French Innovative Leukemia Organisation is aiming at enrolling 50 relapsed/refractory WM patients. Enrollment started in March 2017 and has an estimated primary completion date in March 2019.

Other anti-CD20 monoclonal antibodies, such as veltuzumab and ocrelizumab, are undergoing clinical development, but no WM-specific studies are planned with these agents.

DARATUMUMAB

Daratumumab is a fully human anti-CD38 IgG1k monoclonal antibody. CD38 is a transmembrane glycoprotein with adhesion, receptor, and enzymatic functions and is highly and uniformly expressed in plasma cells. Preclinical studies have shown that daratumumab is a potent inducer of CDC and ADCC in multiple myeloma (MM)-derived cell lines as well as primary MM cells.[34] Of interest, the cell killing effect of daratumumab was not adversely impacted by the presence of bone marrow stromal cells. Additional studies have shown that daratumumab also elicits a potent ADCP in a xenograft mouse model and in primary MM cells, even at variable levels of CD38 expression.[35] Besides CDC, ADCC, and ADCP, daratumumab promotes T-cell expansion, especially helper T cells and cytotoxic T cells, but also depletes immunosuppressive CD38-expressing regulatory T cells, which represents a possible additional mechanism of action for daratumumab.[36] CD38 is highly expressed in the lymphoplasmacytic and plasma cell components of WM, which accounts for 40% to 70% of the WM clone,[7,37] providing a solid argument in favor of the clinical development of anti-CD38 therapy in WM.

Daratumumab is approved by the FDA to treat patients with MM:

- In combination with lenalidomide and dexamethasone, or bortezomib and dexamethasone, for the treatment of patients with MM who have received at least one prior therapy
- In combination with pomalidomide and dexamethasone for the treatment of patients with MM who have received at least 2 prior therapies, including lenalidomide and a proteasome inhibitor
- As monotherapy, for the treatment of patients with MM who have received at least 3 prior lines of therapy, including a proteasome inhibitor and an immunomodulatory agent, or who are double-refractory to a proteasome inhibitor and an immunomodulatory agent

A multicenter prospective phase 2 study evaluating daratumumab in patients with previously treated WM is ongoing (NCT03187262). Daratumumab will be administered at a dose of 16 mg/kg weekly for 8 weeks and then every other week for 16 weeks, followed by 12 monthly infusions. The study aims at enrolling 30 participants. Accrual started in November 2017 with an estimated primary completion date in January 2021.

Other anti-CD38 monoclonal antibodies, such as isatuximab and MOR202, are undergoing clinical development, but no WM-specific studies are planned with these agents.

ULOCUPLUMAB

Ulocuplumab is a fully human anti-CXCR4 monoclonal antibody. The CXCR4 receptor is highly expressed in different hematological malignancies. About 40% of patients with WM can have a mutation in the carboxyl tail of CXCR4.[38] CXCR4 mutations decrease internalization of CXCR4 after CXCL12 binding, promoting constitutive activation of PI3K and ERK, which in turn provides a mechanism of resistance to WM cell killing by alkylators, proteasome inhibitors, and Bruton's Tyrosine Kinase inhibitors.[39] Clinically, WM patients with CXCR4 mutations present with higher levels of serum IgM and symptomatic hyperviscosity. Also, responses to ibrutinib are shorter, more superficial, and of shorter duration in patients with CXCR4 mutations.[40,41]

Ulocuplumab has been shown, in preclinical studies, not only to inhibit CXCR4 activation and migration but also to induce apoptosis of CLL cells at nanomolar concentrations, in the presence or absence of stromal cell support.[42] Ulocuplumab inhibited adhesion of primary MM cells to bone marrow stromal cells and effectively induced anti-MM cell cytotoxicity that was synergistic with bortezomib.[43] A phase 1b study combined ulocuplumab with lenalidomide and dexamethasone or bortezomib and dexamethasone in 44 participants with relapsed/refractory MM and showed evidence of efficacy with an ORR of more than 50%. Thrombocytopenia and anemia were common grade 3 adverse events.[44]

The FDA has not approved ulocuplumab as a treatment of any disease. A phase 1/2 study evaluating the combination of ulocuplumab and ibrutinib in patients with WM is ongoing (NCT03225716). A maximum of 38 participants will be enrolled. Ibrutinib will be given at a dose of 420 mg orally every day. Ulocuplumab will be given at 3 dose levels in a 3 + 3 dose escalation fashion (phase 1) with dose expansion (phase 2) at the highest dose level if no dose-limiting toxicity is observed at lower levels.

Other anti-CXCR4 monoclonal antibodies, such as LY2624587, are undergoing clinical development, but no WM-specific studies are planned with these agents.

OTHER MONOCLONAL ANTIBODIES

Of historical interest is the use of the anti-CD52 monoclonal antibody alemtuzumab in patients with WM. Preclinical studies showed that CD52 was expressed not only in the malignant B cells but also in the bone marrow mast cells of patients with WM.[45,46] A prospective study evaluated alemtuzumab in patients with symptomatic WM.[47] The ORR was 75%; the major response rate was 36%, and the median TTP was 15 months. CMV reactivation occurred, leading to death in 3 patients. Also, late onset autoimmune thrombocytopenia developed in 4 patients and contributed to the death of 1 patient. Alemtuzumab has not been commercialized in the United States and Europe since 2012, but it is currently approved for use in multiple sclerosis.

SUMMARY

For the last 2 decades, anti-CD20 monoclonal antibodies have been the mainstay of therapy for patients with WM. When used in combination with chemotherapy or proteasome inhibitors, the addition of monoclonal antibodies has been associated with higher rates of response as well as PFS. The field is moving beyond anti-CD20 monoclonal antibodies, and novel compounds targeting other membrane markers such as CD38 and CXCR4 are under current clinical development.

REFERENCES

1. Scott AM, Wolchok JD, Old LJ. Antibody therapy of cancer. Nat Rev Cancer 2012; 12(4):278–87.
2. Jaglowski SM, Alinari L, Lapalombella R, et al. The clinical application of monoclonal antibodies in chronic lymphocytic leukemia. Blood 2010;116(19):3705–14.
3. Cartron G, Watier H, Golay J, et al. From the bench to the bedside: ways to improve rituximab efficacy. Blood 2004;104(9):2635–42.
4. Michaud HA, Eliaou JF, Lafont V, et al. Tumor antigen-targeting monoclonal antibody-based immunotherapy: orchestrating combined strategies for the development of long-term antitumor immunity. Oncoimmunology 2014;3(9): e955684.
5. Zhou X, Hu W, Qin X. The role of complement in the mechanism of action of rituximab for B-cell lymphoma: implications for therapy. Oncologist 2008;13(9):954–66.
6. Press OW, Howell-Clark J, Anderson S, et al. Retention of B-cell-specific monoclonal antibodies by human lymphoma cells. Blood 1994;83(5):1390–7.
7. Morice WG, Chen D, Kurtin PJ, et al. Novel immunophenotypic features of marrow lymphoplasmacytic lymphoma and correlation with Waldenstrom's macroglobulinemia. Mod Pathol 2009;22(6):807–16.

8. Olszewski AJ, Treon SP, Castillo JJ. Evolution of management and outcomes in Waldenstrom macroglobulinemia: a population-based analysis. Oncologist 2016;21(11):1377–86.

9. Byrd JC, White CA, Link B, et al. Rituximab therapy in Waldenstrom's macroglobulinemia: preliminary evidence of clinical activity. Ann Oncol 1999;10(12):1525–7.

10. Treon SP, Agus TB, Link B, et al. CD20-directed antibody-mediated immunotherapy induces responses and facilitates hematologic recovery in patients with Waldenstrom's macroglobulinemia. J Immunother 2001;24(3):272–9.

11. Dimopoulos MA, Zervas C, Zomas A, et al. Treatment of Waldenstrom's macroglobulinemia with rituximab. J Clin Oncol 2002;20(9):2327–33.

12. Dimopoulos MA, Zervas C, Zomas A, et al. Extended rituximab therapy for previously untreated patients with Waldenstrom's macroglobulinemia. Clin Lymphoma 2002;3(3):163–6.

13. Treon SP, Emmanouilides C, Kimby E, et al. Extended rituximab therapy in Waldenstrom's macroglobulinemia. Ann Oncol 2005;16(1):132–8.

14. Gertz MA, Rue M, Blood E, et al. Multicenter phase 2 trial of rituximab for Waldenstrom macroglobulinemia (WM): an Eastern Cooperative Oncology Group Study (E3A98). Leuk Lymphoma 2004;45(10):2047–55.

15. Ghobrial IM, Fonseca R, Greipp PR, et al. Initial immunoglobulin M 'flare' after rituximab therapy in patients diagnosed with Waldenstrom macroglobulinemia: an Eastern Cooperative Oncology Group Study. Cancer 2004;101(11):2593–8.

16. Treon SP, Branagan AR, Hunter Z, et al. Paradoxical increases in serum IgM and viscosity levels following rituximab in Waldenstrom's macroglobulinemia. Ann Oncol 2004;15(10):1481–3.

17. Leblond V, Kastritis E, Advani R, et al. Treatment recommendations from the Eighth International Workshop on Waldenstrom's Macroglobulinemia. Blood 2016;128(10):1321–8.

18. Treon SP, Soumerai JD, Branagan AR, et al. Thalidomide and rituximab in Waldenstrom macroglobulinemia. Blood 2008;112(12):4452–7.

19. Treon SP, Soumerai JD, Branagan AR, et al. Lenalidomide and rituximab in Waldenstrom's macroglobulinemia. Clin Cancer Res 2009;15(1):355–60.

20. Treon SP, Hanzis C, Manning RJ, et al. Maintenance Rituximab is associated with improved clinical outcome in rituximab naive patients with Waldenstrom Macroglobulinaemia who respond to a rituximab-containing regimen. Br J Haematol 2011;154(3):357–62.

21. Castillo JJ, Gustine JN, Meid K, et al. Response and survival for primary therapy combination regimens and maintenance rituximab in Waldenstrom macroglobulinaemia. Br J Haematol 2018;181(1):77–85.

22. Teeling JL, Mackus WJ, Wiegman LJ, et al. The biological activity of human CD20 monoclonal antibodies is linked to unique epitopes on CD20. J Immunol 2006; 177(1):362–71.

23. Teeling JL, French RR, Cragg MS, et al. Characterization of new human CD20 monoclonal antibodies with potent cytolytic activity against non-Hodgkin lymphomas. Blood 2004;104(6):1793–800.

24. Golay J, Zaffaroni L, Vaccari T, et al. Biologic response of B lymphoma cells to anti-CD20 monoclonal antibody rituximab in vitro: CD55 and CD59 regulate complement-mediated cell lysis. Blood 2000;95(12):3900–8.

25. Furman RR, Eradat HA, DiRienzo CG, et al. Once-weekly ofatumumab in untreated or relapsed Waldenstrom's macroglobulinaemia: an open-label, single-arm, phase 2 study. Lancet Haematol 2017;4(1):e24–34.

26. Gavriatopoulou M, Kastritis E, Kyrtsonis MC, et al. Phase 2 study of ofatumumab, fludarabine and cyclophosphamide in relapsed/refractory Waldenstrom's macroglobulinemia. Leuk Lymphoma 2017;58(6):1506–8.

27. Treon SP, Hanzis C, Tripsas C, et al. Bendamustine therapy in patients with relapsed or refractory Waldenstrom's macroglobulinemia. Clin Lymphoma Myeloma Leuk 2011;11(1):133–5.

28. Castillo JJ, Kanan S, Meid K, et al. Rituximab intolerance in patients with Waldenstrom macroglobulinaemia. Br J Haematol 2016;174(4):645–8.

29. Niederfellner G, Lammens A, Mundigl O, et al. Epitope characterization and crystal structure of GA101 provide insights into the molecular basis for type I/II distinction of CD20 antibodies. Blood 2011;118(2):358–67.

30. Mossner E, Brunker P, Moser S, et al. Increasing the efficacy of CD20 antibody therapy through the engineering of a new type II anti-CD20 antibody with enhanced direct and immune effector cell-mediated B-cell cytotoxicity. Blood 2010;115(22):4393–402.

31. Terszowski G, Klein C, Stern M. KIR/HLA interactions negatively affect rituximab-but not GA101 (obinutuzumab)-induced antibody-dependent cellular cytotoxicity. J Immunol 2014;192(12):5618–24.

32. Herter S, Birk MC, Klein C, et al. Glycoengineering of therapeutic antibodies enhances monocyte/macrophage-mediated phagocytosis and cytotoxicity. J Immunol 2014;192(5):2252–60.

33. Herter S, Herting F, Mundigl O, et al. Preclinical activity of the type II CD20 antibody GA101 (obinutuzumab) compared with rituximab and ofatumumab in vitro and in xenograft models. Mol Cancer Ther 2013;12(10):2031–42.

34. de Weers M, Tai YT, van der Veer MS, et al. Daratumumab, a novel therapeutic human CD38 monoclonal antibody, induces killing of multiple myeloma and other hematological tumors. J Immunol 2011;186(3):1840–8.

35. Overdijk MB, Verploegen S, Bogels M, et al. Antibody-mediated phagocytosis contributes to the anti-tumor activity of the therapeutic antibody daratumumab in lymphoma and multiple myeloma. MAbs 2015;7(2):311–21.

36. Krejcik J, Casneuf T, Nijhof IS, et al. Daratumumab depletes CD38+ immune regulatory cells, promotes T-cell expansion, and skews T-cell repertoire in multiple myeloma. Blood 2016;128(3):384–94.

37. Konoplev S, Medeiros LJ, Bueso-Ramos CE, et al. Immunophenotypic profile of lymphoplasmacytic lymphoma/Waldenstrom macroglobulinemia. Am J Clin Pathol 2005;124(3):414–20.

38. Hunter ZR, Xu L, Yang G, et al. The genomic landscape of Waldenstrom macroglobulinemia is characterized by highly recurring MYD88 and WHIM-like CXCR4 mutations, and small somatic deletions associated with B-cell lymphomagenesis. Blood 2014;123(11):1637–46.

39. Cao Y, Hunter ZR, Liu X, et al. CXCR4 WHIM-like frameshift and nonsense mutations promote ibrutinib resistance but do not supplant MYD88(L265P) -directed survival signalling in Waldenstrom macroglobulinaemia cells. Br J Haematol 2015;168(5):701–7.

40. Treon SP, Meid K, Gustine J, et al. Long-term follow-up of previously treated patients who received ibrutinib for symptomatic Waldenstrom's macroglobulinemia: update of pivotal clinical trial. Blood 2017;130(Suppl 1):2766.

41. Treon SP, Tripsas CK, Meid K, et al. Ibrutinib in previously treated Waldenstrom's macroglobulinemia. N Engl J Med 2015;372(15):1430–40.

42. Kashyap MK, Kumar D, Jones H, et al. Ulocuplumab (BMS-936564/MDX1338): a fully human anti-CXCR4 antibody induces cell death in chronic lymphocytic

leukemia mediated through a reactive oxygen species-dependent pathway. On-cotarget 2016;7(3):2809–22.

43. Roccaro AM, Sacco A, Kuhne M, et al. The new CXCR4 inhibitor MDX-1338 exerts anti-tumor activity in multiple myeloma. Blood 2011;118(21):1844.

44. Ghobrial IM, Perez R, Baz R, et al. Phase Ib study of the novel anti-CXCR4 antibody ulocuplumab (BMS-936564) in combination with lenalidomide plus low-dose dexamethasone, or with bortezomib plus dexamethasone in subjects with relapsed or refractory multiple myeloma. Blood 2014;124(21):3483.

45. Owen RG, Hillmen P, Rawstron AC. CD52 expression in Waldenstrom's macro-globulinemia: implications for alemtuzumab therapy and response assessment. Clin Lymphoma 2005;5(4):278–81.

46. Santos DD, Hatjiharissi E, Tournilhac O, et al. CD52 is expressed on human mast cells and is a potential therapeutic target in Waldenstrom's Macroglobulinemia and mast cell disorders. Clin Lymphoma Myeloma 2006;6(6):478–83.

47. Treon SP, Soumerai JD, Hunter ZR, et al. Long-term follow-up of symptomatic patients with lymphoplasmacytic lymphoma/Waldenstrom macroglobulinemia treated with the anti-CD52 monoclonal antibody alemtuzumab. Blood 2011;118(2):276–81.

48. Dimopoulos MA, Anagnostopoulos A, Kyrtsonis MC, et al. Primary treatment of Waldenstrom macroglobulinemia with dexamethasone, rituximab, and cyclo-phosphamide. J Clin Oncol 2007;25(22):3344–9.

49. Buske C, Hoster E, Dreyling M, et al. The addition of rituximab to front-line therapy with CHOP (R-CHOP) results in a higher response rate and longer time to treatment failure in patients with lymphoplasmacytic lymphoma: results of a randomized trial of the German Low-Grade Lymphoma Study Group (GLSG). Leukemia 2009;23(1):153–61.

50. Treon SP, Branagan AR, Ioakimidis L, et al. Long-term outcomes to fludarabine and rituximab in Waldenstrom macroglobulinemia. Blood 2009;113(16):3673–8.

51. Tedeschi A, Benevolo G, Varettoni M, et al. Fludarabine plus cyclophosphamide and rituximab in Waldenstrom macroglobulinemia: an effective but myelosup-pressive regimen to be offered to patients with advanced disease. Cancer 2012;118(2):434–43.

52. Rummel MJ, Niederle N, Maschmeyer G, et al. Bendamustine plus rituximab versus CHOP plus rituximab as first-line treatment for patients with indolent and mantle-cell lymphomas: an open-label, multicentre, randomised, phase 3 non-inferiority trial. Lancet 2013;381(9873):1203–10.

53. Treon SP, Ioakimidis L, Soumerai JD, et al. Primary therapy of Waldenstrom macroglobulinemia with bortezomib, dexamethasone, and rituximab: WMCTG clinical trial 05-180. J Clin Oncol 2009;27(23):3830–5.

54. Dimopoulos MA, Garcia-Sanz R, Gavriatopoulou M, et al. Primary therapy of Waldenstrom macroglobulinemia (WM) with weekly bortezomib, low-dose dexamethasone, and rituximab (BDR): long-term results of a phase 2 study of the European Myeloma Network (EMN). Blood 2013;122(19):3276–82.

55. Treon SP, Tripsas CK, Meid K, et al. Carfilzomib, rituximab, and dexamethasone (CaRD) treatment offers a neuropathy-sparing approach for treating Waldenstrom's macroglobulinemia. Blood 2014;124(4):503–10.

56. Castillo JJ, Meid K, Gustine J, et al. Prospective clinical trial of ixazomib, dexamethasone and rituximab as primary therapy in Waldenström macroglobulinemia. Clin Cancer Res 2018. [Epub ahead of print].

First-Generation and Second-Generation Bruton Tyrosine Kinase Inhibitors in Waldenström Macroglobulinemia

Kimon V. Argyropoulos, MD[a], M. Lia, MD[b],*

KEYWORDS

- Waldenström macroglobulinemia • BTK • Ibrutinib
- Second-generation BTK inhibitors

KEY POINTS

- Constitutive Bruton tyrosine kinase (BTK) activation is a significant factor for the pathogenesis of Waldenström macroglobulinemia.
- Ibrutinib is a first-generation BTK inhibitor, which is approved by the Food and Drug Administration and European Medicines Agency for the management of symptomatic Waldenström macroglobulinemia and provides durable and deep responses.
- The occurrence of resistance and the adverse events related to ibrutinib have led to the development of novel and more specific BTK inhibitors, which are currently evaluated for their efficacy and safety in clinical studies.

INTRODUCTION

Waldenström macroglobulinemia (WM) is an indolent B-cell non-Hodgkin lymphoma characterized by the accumulation of IgM-secreting clonal lymphoplasmacytic cells in the bone marrow and often in extramedullary sites, including the spleen. After an extensive characterization of the genomic landscape in WM, MYD88 L265P (>90% of cases) and CXCR4–warts, hypogammaglobulinemia, infections, and myelokathexis (WHIM)-like mutations (30%–40% of cases) have emerged as the pathologic hallmarks of the disease, proving the significance of these 2 signaling axes in the pathobiology of WM.[1-3] B-cell receptor (BCR) signaling-associated mutations occur less

Disclosure Statement: The authors have no relationship with a commercial company that has a direct financial interest in subject matter or materials discussed in article or with a company making a competing product.
a Immunology Program, Memorial Sloan Kettering Cancer Center, 408 East 69th Street, New York, NY 10021, USA; b Department of Medicine, Lymphoma Service, Memorial Sloan Kettering Cancer Center, 1275 York Avenue, New York, NY 10065, USA
* Corresponding author.
E-mail address: Palombam@mskcc.org

frequently and are restricted to the CD79A and CD79B genes, in approximately 15% of WM cases.[2,4] Evidence for BCR utilization stems from immunoglobulin heavy-chain variable region gene (IGHV) sequencing studies, however, which show the presence of a high mutational load and skewed repertoire, and functional BCR signaling studies in WM cells, which show hyperactivation of the BCR signalosome.[5–8]

From a therapeutic standpoint, because malignant transformation in WM occurs in the context of aberrant and complex signaling networks, it is important to identify targets that operate downstream of multiple signaling pathways. Among most intracellular signaling kinases, Bruton tyrosine kinase (BTK) has been shown to participate as a central node in multiple signaling pathways that are biologically active in WM.[7,9] Moreover, BTK is the target of several novel small molecule compounds that show high clinical activity in WM patients. Given the biological and clinical significance of the BTK protein, this review summarizes the function of BTK in WM cells and presents current preclinical and clinical knowledge on the first-in-class, irreversible BTK inhibitor, ibrutinib, and the new generation of BTK inhibitors.

BRUTON TYROSINE KINASE AND ITS SIGNIFICANCE FOR WALDENSTRÖM MACROGLOBULINEMIA CELL BIOLOGY

BTK was discovered in 1993 and was named after Ogden Bruton, who first described the primary immunodeficiency X-linked agammaglobulinemia syndrome, resulting from germline mutations in the BTK gene.[10–12] BTK is crucial for normal B-cell development in the bone marrow after the pre–B-cell stage, whereas in mature, peripheral B cells, BTK activation promotes cell activation, proliferation, and survival.[13–15] BTK was initially described as pre-BCR and BCR-dependent kinase[16–18] that phosphorylates PLCγ2, resulting in increased phospholipase activity, subsequently resulting in the activation of distal signaling effectors, including extracellular-signal-regulated kinase (ERK) and nuclear factor (NF)-κB.[18–20] It was soon discovered, however, that multiple receptors in a B cell can activate this kinase. Of particular significance was the discovery that BTK is a functional element of TLR/MYD88 signaling, suggesting that the phosphorylation of this protein is significant for the propagation of both adaptive and innate receptor-mediated signals.[21,22] In addition to the TLR pathway, BTK is a protein involved in the signaling propagation of many G-coupled chemokine receptors.[23]

BTK expression is maintained in many B-cell leukemias and lymphomas; therefore, after its discovery, BTK became an attractive therapeutic target.[24] The first small molecule targeting BTK was LFM-A13, which showed significant in vitro antileukemic activity.[25] Following that example, multiple more specific inhibitors were developed, including ibrutinib, which showed significant antilymphoma activity in autochthonous canine B-cell lymphomas.[26] In human lymphomas, the first evidence of BTK activation and its role in oncogenic BCR signaling was highlighted in the activated B-cell–like subtype of diffuse large B-cell lymphoma.[27] BTK activation in WM was first described as an epiphenomenon of the MYD88 L265P mutation. Coimmunoprecipitation experiments revealed that BTK complexes with MYD88 in L265P-mutated WM cells, whereas mutated cells exhibit significantly higher BTK phosphorylation compared with MYD88 wild-type cells. In this study, BTK inhibition abrogated the binding of BTK to the mutant MYD88 protein, mitigated NF-κB activation, and resulted in significant WM cell death in vitro.[9] This seminal work by Yang and colleagues[9] was the first to provide a molecular link between MYD88 mutations and NF-κB activation in WM and highlighted the need for the clinical assessment of ibrutinib in WM patients. The authors' group analyzed BCR signaling activation in primary WM samples, using multiparametric phospho-flow cytometry and assessed the levels of all phosphoproteins comprising the BCR signalosome, including BTK. WM B cells showed striking features of chronic active BCR signaling yet with remarkable heterogeneity among patients. The signaling potential through the BCR in WM cells correlated with high levels of surface IgM expression but not with the BCR mutation status of these patients (neither IGHV mutation load nor CD79A/B mutations), proving that increased pathway activity can arise in the absence of signaling-associated genetic alterations. Patient-specific phosphosignatures revealed, however, that heightened BCR activity correlated with patients experiencing a more aggressive disease course compared with patients with healthy-like BCR activity, who on the contrary were more likely to have stable disease. In the authors' study, although BTK was a functional member of the BCR signalosome and WM cells exhibited more prolonged kinetics of BTK phosphorylation compared with normal B cells, BTK inhibition prior to BCR stimulation only partially inhibited PLCγ2 phosphorylation, and WM cells were less sensitive to apoptosis induction compared with inhibition of more proximal kinases, such as SYK and Src. This suggested that complete BCR signaling inhibition occurs at the very proximal kinase level and BTK might be partially bypassed in the context of BCR signaling.[7] In agreement with these findings, de Rooij and colleagues[28,29] showed that ibrutinib shows inferior cytotoxic activity compared with idelalisib in WM cell lines; nonetheless, ibrutinib inhibited BCR-induced, integrin-mediated cell adhesion, suggesting that BTK inhibition results in poor retention of WM cells in lymphoid organs and subsequent death in the absence of a protective microenvironment. The investigators did not notice any ibrutinib effects on CXCR4-induced, integrin-mediated adhesion, suggesting that the role of BTK is redundant in CXCR4-mediated adhesion. Inversely, BTK inhibition has been shown to down-regulate CXCR4 expression in malignant B cells.[30] These findings are on par with the clinical effects of ibrutinib, which results in rapid lymphocytosis in most MYD88-mutated/CXCR4–wild type (WT) patients and a delayed responsiveness in MYD88-mutated/CXCR4-WHIM–mutated patients, who exhibit persistent CXCR4 membrane expression and sustained CXCR4 signaling.[31,32]

In addition to the WM cell-intrinsic effects, discussed previously, ibrutinib has immunomodulatory properties. Although T cells are the only hematopoietic subsets that do not express BTK, ibrutinib has been shown to bind and irreversibly inhibit inducible T-cell kinase (ITK), which is the T-cell homolog of BTK. ITK inhibition by ibrutinib results in significant TCR signaling abrogation, protects T_H1-CD4$^+$ and cytotoxic CD8$^+$ T cells, and promotes generalized T_H1 skewing in vitro and in vivo.[33] BTK is also expressed by the monocytic lineage as a member of the TLR signaling pathway. Ibrutinib was recently shown to attenuate the secretion of homeostatic chemokines by tumor-associated macrophages, resulting in compromised adhesion and invasion of lymphoid malignant cells. Moreover, ibrutinib-treated macrophages have an impaired capacity to secrete angiogenic cytokines and promote angiogenesis.[34]

THE CLINICAL EXPERIENCE WITH IBRUTINIB AND NOVEL BRUTON TYROSINE KINASE INHIBITORS IN WALDENSTRÖM MACROGLOBULINEMIA

Ibrutinib

Ibrutinib is a first-generation irreversible BTK inhibitor and first drug to be approved for WM by the United States Food and Drug Administration (FDA) and the European Medicines Agency (EMA). The approval of ibrutinib was supported by a pivotal phase 2 clinical trial in 63 refractory or relapsed WM patients, published by Treon and colleagues in 2015.[31] A long term follow-up of this study was recently presented at the

59th American Society of Hematology annual meeting.[35] Patients received oral ibrutinib, 420 mg daily (protocol administered ibrutinib for 40 months and commercial supply thereafter). The median time on ibrutinib was 46.6 months (range 0.5–60 months). Long-term results showed an overall response rate of 90.5%, comprised of 27% very good partial responders. Major response rate was 77.7%, which is the highest achieved so far in a cohort of refractory or relapsed WM patients compared with rituximab (20%) or bortezomib regimen (48%).[36,37] At time of best response, median IgM levels decreased from 3520 mg/dL to 821 mg/dL, median hemoglobin increased from 10.5 g/dL to 14.2 g/dL, and median bone marrow involvement decreased from 60% to 20%. Response rates to ibrutinib differed significantly based on patients' genotype, with the highest rates of major responses observed in MYD88-mutated/CXCR4-WT patients (97.2%), followed by MYD88-mutated/CXCR4-WHIM–mutated patients (66.6%). No major responses were observed in MYD88-WT/CXCR4-WT patients (0%), although this genotype is rare (n = 5). Ibrutinib results in rapid responses with a median time to response of 4 weeks. Median time to major responses are seen in MYD88-mutated/CXCR4-WT patients within 2 months of treatment (range 1–49 months), but in MYD88-mutated/CXCR4-WHIM–mutated patients they are seen within 6 months of therapy (range 1–40 months). With a median study follow-up of 47.1 months, the median progression-free survival (PFS) for MYD88-mutated/CXCR4-WT was not reached, yet the median PFS was 45 months for MYD88-mutated/CXCR4-WHIM–mutated patients, and 21 months for MYD88-WT/CXCR4-WT patients. Although the population of refractory/relapsed patients in the study, discussed previously, was heterogeneous in terms of prior treatment history (monoclonal antibodies, proteasome inhibitors, alkylating agents, and nucleoside analogs), response rates to ibrutinib were not impacted by the nature of the prior agents used. In the recently published arm C of the multicenter iNNOVATE study by Dimopoulos and colleagues,[38] a homogeneous population of 31 rituximab refractory patients were treated with oral ibrutinib, 420 mg daily, and followed prospectively for safety and efficacy (median follow-up was 18.1 months). The study similarly showed sustained responses and manageable toxicity, achieving an overall response rate of 90%, major response rate of 71%, and an estimated 18-month PFS rate of 86% and overall survival rate of 97%.

Although the activity of ibrutinib in previously untreated individuals was until recently unknown, a new phase II clinical trial investigated the effects of the drug in this population. Data from 30 treatment-naive, symptomatic WM patients presented by Treon and colleagues[39] at the 59th American Society of Hematology annual meeting showed overall and major response rates of 96.7% and 80%, respectively; 17% of the patients achieved a very good partial response (VGPR). At best response, serum IgM declined from a median of 4380 to 1786, median bone marrow involvement declined from 65% to 20%, and median hemoglobin level increased from 10.3 g/dL to 13.6 g/dL. Lymphadenopathy (n = 7 [70%]) and splenomegaly (n = 4 [80%]) decreased or resolved in most patients with baseline extramedullary disease.

In no clinical trial has ibrutinib treatment resulted in complete remission, which suggests an inherent, partial resistance of WM clones to BTK inhibition. Signaling studies of primary WM cells in patients receiving ibrutinib treatment reveal suppressed BTK activity, yet IRAK1 and IRAK4 remain phosphorylated and transduce NF-κB–mediated survival signals.[40] Moreover, as discussed previously, although BTK is a central node in the BCR signalosome, it can be bypassed by more proximal kinases, like SYK and Src kinases, which can directly activate more downstream proteins, like PLCγ2.[7] These findings suggest that a combination of ibrutinib with IRAK, SYK, or Src kinase inhibitors might be more potent to induce a complete remission. Meanwhile, acquired resistance to ibrutinib therapy has emerged in multiple B-cell lymphomas treated with ibrutinib.[41] Half of the WM patients that progress on ibrutinib acquire new mutations on the BTK gene on cysteine 481, which abrogates the binding of the drug to the protein, while it mediates novel routes of cell survival through sustained ERK phosphorylation and proinflammatory cytokine secretion.[42,43] Furthermore, PLCγ2 and CARD11 mutations described in ibrutinib-resistant B-cell lymphomas have also been identified in ibrutinib-resistant WM patients.[42]

Given these inherent and acquired mechanisms of signaling resistance, the next approach would be to combine ibrutinib with other active agents, which act on non–signaling-related WM biological features. Arms A and B of the iNNOVATE phase 3 clinical study currently examine the combination of rituximab with ibrutinib versus rituximab with placebo (NCT02165397). Because there is a significant CD20$^-$ plasma cell fraction of WM clones that is resistant to rituximab, it would be interesting to evaluate the synergistic potential of agents that can target plasma cells, like the anti-CD38 antibody daratumumab, whose activity is currently being assessed in the context of a phase 2 clinical trial in previously treated WM patients (NCT03187262).[44] From a different mechanistic standpoint, BCL-2 is known to inhibit ibrutinib's cytotoxic activity in WM cells and the BCL-2 antagonist venetoclax has resulted in major clinical responses in 4 WM patients in a phase 1 study.[45,46] Currently, a clinical trial examines venetoclax in previously treated WM patients (NCT02677324) and is expected to support further studies on the combination of venetoclax with ibrutinib in WM. Finally, because a patient's genotype is one of the most crucial factors to be taken into consideration during the design of new clinical trials in WM, the unique biology and clinical behavior of CXCR4-WHIM–mutated WM patients has successfully led to a new clinical trial investigating the combination of the CXCR4-blocking antibody ulocuplumab with ibrutinib in CXCR4-WHIM–mutated WM patients (NCT03225716).

Although ibrutinib is well tolerated and induces deep and durable responses against symptomatic treatment-naive and refractory/relapsed WM, it has substantial toxicities. The most common grades 3 to 4 adverse events in WM include neutropenia (15%) and thrombocytopenia (13%), anemia, atrial fibrillation (AF), pneumonia, endocarditis, herpes zoster, urinary tract infection, subcutaneous abscess, hematoma, and syncope (2% for each).[31] In the absence of complete remissions, ibrutinib maintenance treatment is essential; therefore, the emergence of adverse events is a management challenge. It is important to highlight that withholding or discontinuing ibrutinib can lead to rapid increases in serum IgM, decrease in hemoglobin and re-emergence of symptomatology compared with other regimens that have a slower post-treatment disease recurrence. Despite their low occurrence, hemorrhage and AF have been encountered in most clinical studies and raise concerns for the management of these patients. A recently published meta-analysis of published randomized trials showed that the overall bleeding relative risk is significantly higher in patients receiving ibrutinib; nonetheless, the major bleeding relative risk is not statistically significant.[47] Similarly, a meta-analysis of published randomized trials showed a statistically significant risk for AF in patients receiving ibrutinib.[48] Overall, ibrutinib-related adverse events are considered to occur due to binding to other TEC kinases and members of the epidermal growth factor receptor (EGFR) family.[26] Nevertheless, it is still not fully elucidated which of the reported side effects are due to on-target BTK inhibition in nonlymphoma tissues or off-target kinase inhibition. In regard to bleeding, in vitro and ex vivo studies show that ibrutinib affects collagen and von Willebrand factor–induced platelet aggregation, secondary to BTK/TEC kinase inhibition in platelets.[49,50] Moreover, ibrutinib inhibits Src family kinases, resulting in the formation of unstable thrombi.[51] The pathophysiology of ibrutinib-induced AF is still not fully understood, although there is evidence of higher BTK/TEC expression in the myocardium of AF patients compared with patients with sinus rhythm, whereas ibrutinib seems to inhibit the transduction of cardioprotective PI3K/AKT signaling.[52]

Novel Bruton Tyrosine Kinase Inhibitors

The occurrence of resistance and the adverse events related to ibrutinib have led to the development of novel more specific BTK inhibitors, such as zanubrutinib (BGB-3111), ONO/GS-4059, acalabrutinib (ACP-196), and vecabrutinib (SNS-062), which are currently evaluated for their efficacy and safety in clinical studies.

Zanubrutinib (BGB-3111)

Zanubrutinib is a highly bioavailable, irreversible BTK inhibitor. It is equipotent to ibrutinib in regard to BTK inhibition, yet it exhibits highly superior selectivity for BTK, relative to similar tyrosine kinases, including ITK, TEC, EGFR, HER2, and JAK3. Zanubrutinib's half maximal inhibitory concentration (IC-50) values for these off-target kinases were 2-fold to 70-fold higher compared with ibrutinib, predicting less toxicity at the same concentrations in vivo.[53,54] Due to the weaker activity on ITK, zanubrutinib has been reported to be significantly weaker compared with ibrutinib in inhibiting rituximab-induced antibody-mediated cytotoxicity.[53] Moreover, in B-cell lymphoma xenograft models, zanubrutinib induced dose-dependent antitumor effects and had superior efficacy compared with ibrutinib.[53] Ibrutinib shows borderline target inhibition in peripheral blood, whereas preclinical models have shown a significant recovery of BTK occupancy in hematopoietic tissues within 24-hour postibrutinib administration.[55] In humans, an open-label phase 1 trial of zanubrutinib as a modified 3 + 3 dose-escalation design (40 mg, 80 mg, 160 mg, and 320 mg orally every day and 160 mg orally twice a day) in patients with B-cell lymphomas has shown that complete BTK occupancy is achieved in peripheral blood mononuclear cells at a starting dose of 40 mg. Moreover, paired lymph node biopsies show 100% median trough occupancy at 160 mg twice daily versus 94% median trough occupancy when given at 320 mg once daily.[54]

Results from a phase 1 clinical study in WM patients with zanubrutinib were presented at the 2017 International Conference on Malignant Lymphoma biennial by Trotman and colleagues.[56] The study included 42 WM patients evaluable for efficacy, 33 of whom were refractory/relapsed and 9 were treatment-naive. Median age was 66 years old and the median follow-up was 10.6 months. Zanubrutinib was tolerable and highly active, with a best objective response rate of 90% and a major response rate of 76%. VGPR rate was 43%, which is superior to the VGPR rate achieved by ibrutinib (27%). Partial response rate was 33% and minor response rate was 14%. No complete response was achieved. At time of best response, median IgM levels decreased from 3270 mg/dL to 610 mg/dL, median hemoglobin increased from 10.45 g/dL to 14.2 g/dL, and median lymphadenopathy by CT showed a 45% median reduction. The 1-year PFS was 91.7%. The most common grade 1 to grade 2 adverse events reported in at least 20% of patients included petechiae/purpura/contusion (35%), upper respiratory infections (31%), and constipation (25%). The most frequent grade 3 or grade 4 events included anemia (8%) and neutropenia (8%). Serious hemorrhage ($\geq$grade 3) occurred in 1 patient (2%). AF occurred in 3 patients (6%), yet no greater than or equal to grade 3 AF was reported. A phase 3, randomized clinical study comparing the efficacy and safety of zanubrutinib (160 mg orally twice a day, arm A) and ibrutinib (420 mg orally every day, arm B) in WM is currently ongoing, but no results have yet been reported (NCT03053440).

ONO/GS-4059

ONO/GS-4059 is a highly selective, irreversible BTK inhibitor. The first-in-human phase 1, dose-escalation study of ONO/GS-4059 was on a broad range of relapsed/refractory B-cell lymphomas.[57] There were 9 dose-escalation groups ranging from 20 mg to 600 mg once daily with twice-daily regimen of 240 mg and 300 mg. The pharmacokinetics of ONO/GS-4059 showed rapid absorption and elimination with maximal plasma concentration reached between 2 hours and 3 hours postdose and a half-life of 6.5 hours to 8 hours. ONO/GS-4059 was well tolerated and remarkably efficacious against chronic lymphocytic leukemia (CLL) patients, with an overall response rate of 96%, and mantle cell lymphoma (MCL) patients, with an overall response rate of 92%. WM patients in this study were only 3. In 2 of 3 patients, ONO/GS-4059 was discontinued and in 1 patient a partial response was achieved. In this study, a grade 3 spontaneous muscle hematoma occurred in 1 patient. Five patients developed AF during the study, although in 4 of 5 patients it preexisted and in the other it occurred in the context of pneumonia. Overall, ONO/GS-4059 has a favorable safety profile and a high efficacy in patients with relapsed/refractory B cell malignancies, but its specific profile against WM has to be further investigated.

Acalabrutinib (ACP-196)

Acalabrutinib is an irreversible and selective BTK inhibitor, which shows no activity against ITK and EGFR family proteins, as shown in biochemical assays and functional assays in T cells and natural killer cells (ITK) and lung epithelial cells (EGFR).[58] Among all second-generation BTK inhibitors, acalabrutinib is in the most advanced stages of clinical development. In a pivotal phase 1/2 clinical study acalabrutinib demonstrated high efficacy in patients with refractory/relapsed CLL, with an overall response rate of 95%, including 100% response rate in patients harboring del(17)p.[59] Acalabrutinib had a good tolerability and low occurrence of adverse events, mostly grade 1 or grade 2, with no cases of AF or major bleeding events. Transient headaches occurred more frequently than with ibrutinib. The efficacy of acalabrutinib in MCL patients was recently presented in the 59th American Society of Hematology annual meeting, showing an 81% overall response rate and a 40% complete remission rate, resulting to an accelerated FDA approval of acalabrutinib for MCL, with at least 1 prior therapy.[60] A phase 2 study is currently evaluating the safety and efficacy of acalabrutinib in WM patients (NCT02180724).

Vecabrutinib (SNS-062)

Vecabrutinib is the only noncovalent second-generation BTK inhibitor. Like all second-generation inhibitors, it has a restricted kinase inhibition profile. The unique feature of this drug is that, as opposed to ibrutinib and acalabrutinib, it is active against both WT BTK and C481S-mutated BTK, rendering it a good candidate for patients carrying BTK C481S mutations that develop ibrutinib resistance.[61] In a phase 1a, single-dose clinical study on normal human subjects, vecabrutinib exhibited favorable bioavailability, with rapid absorption and higher mean concentrations achieved at the lowest dose of 50 mg, exceeding those reported for ibrutinib, at 420 mg every day, and acalabrutinib, 100 mg twice a day. Vecabrutinib also demonstrated rapid and near complete pBTK inhibition at all doses.[62] A phase 1b study is under way in patients with B-cell malignancies with and without the BTK C481S mutation (NCT03037645).

Ibrutinib Discontinuation

Temporary treatment interruption is sometimes required in patient receiving ibrutinib.[63] Common causes of drug interruption are management of toxicities or surgical procedures. Most patients who hold ibrutinib experience a mild trend in increased

IgM and decreased hemoglobin, with only approximately a third of the patient meeting criteria for progression of disease. Furthermore, approximately one-fifth of the patients who hold ibrutinib experience withdrawal symptoms consisting of fever and chills, body aches, and arthralgia, possibly due to the re-emergence of proinflammatory cytokines, which had been kept in check during ibrutinib therapy. Steroids were used successfully to mitigate the withdrawal symptoms. Generally, resuming ibrutinib results in resolution of symptoms and response of any sign of progression within weeks. A study of disease outcome was recently conducted on 51 of 189 patients treated with ibrutinib who needed to permanently discontinue therapy due to progression toxicity or no response.[64] The study revealed that patients with CXCR4 mutations are more likely to discontinue therapy and that abrupt IgM rebound after ibrutinib discontinuation was associated with IgM-related morbidity and worse response to salvage therapy. If clinically possible, continuation of ibrutinib until next therapy should be considered.

SUMMARY

Ibrutinib is currently the only FDA-approved and EMA-approved medication for symptomatic WM, and its durable and deep responses have radically changed the management of WM patients. Nevertheless the emergence of mutations that confer ibrutinib resistance and the toxicity of the drug, have dictated the development of second-generation BTK inhibitors. These novel inhibitors are more selective for BTK, which can result in a lower incidence of adverse events. Given the need for indefinite, continuous treatment, fewer adverse events might result in fewer treatment discontinuations and PFS prolongation in WM patients. Moreover, new inhibitors, like vecabrutinib, could overcome acquired BTK C481S-induced resistance to ibrutinib, although it would not be expected to overcome PLCγ2-induced and CARD11-mutation–induced resistance. Most importantly it is unclear whether any novel BTK inhibitor can induce complete remissions in WM patients, because WM clones inherently exploit alternative signaling routes to escape BTK inhibition. Therefore, a combinatorial approach, including agents like venetoclax, monoclonal antibodies, or chemotherapeutic agents, could target different aspects of WM cell biology and result in superior clinical responses compared with BTK inhibitor monotherapy.

REFERENCES

1. Treon SP, Xu L, Yang G, et al. MYD88 L265P somatic mutation in Waldenstrom's macroglobulinemia. N Engl J Med 2012;367:826–33.
2. Hunter ZR, Xu L, Yang G, et al. The genomic landscape of Waldenstrom macroglobulinemia is characterized by highly recurring MYD88 and WHIM-like CXCR4 mutations, and small somatic deletions associated with B-cell lymphomagenesis. Blood 2014;123:1637–46.
3. Roccaro AM, Sacco A, Jimenez C, et al. C1013G/CXCR4 acts as a driver mutation of tumor progression and modulator of drug resistance in lymphoplasmacytic lymphoma. Blood 2014;123:4120–31.
4. Poulain S, Roumier C, Galiegue-Zouitina S, et al. Genome wide SNP array identified multiple mechanisms of genetic changes in Waldenstrom macroglobulinemia. Am J Hematol 2013;88:948–54.
5. Varettoni M, Zibellini S, Capello D, et al. Clues to pathogenesis of Waldenstrom macroglobulinemia and immunoglobulin M monoclonal gammopathy of undetermined significance provided by analysis of immunoglobulin heavy chain gene

rearrangement and clustering of B-cell receptors. Leuk Lymphoma 2013;54: 2485–9.

6. Petrikkos L, Kyrtsonis MC, Roumelioti M, et al. Clonotypic analysis of immuno-globulin heavy chain sequences in patients with Waldenstrom's macroglobuli-nemia: correlation with MYD88 L265P somatic mutation status, clinical features, and outcome. Biomed Res Int 2014;2014:809103.

7. Argyropoulos KV, Vogel R, Ziegler C, et al. Clonal B cells in Waldenstrom's macro-globulinemia exhibit functional features of chronic active B-cell receptor signaling. Leukemia 2016;30:1116–25.

8. Munshi M, LX, Chen J, et al: Mutated MYD88 activates the BCR component SYK and provides a rationale therapeutic target in Waldenstrom's Macroglobulinemia. Presented at the 59th ASH meeting. Atlanta, GA, December, 2017.

9. Yang G, Zhou Y, Liu X, et al. A mutation in MYD88 (L265P) supports the survival of lymphoplasmacytic cells by activation of Bruton tyrosine kinase in Waldenstrom macroglobulinemia. Blood 2013;122:1222–32.

10. Bruton OC. Agammaglobulinemia. Pediatrics 1952;9:722–8.

11. Thomas JD, Sideras P, Smith CI, et al. Colocalization of X-linked agammaglobu-linemia and X-linked immunodeficiency genes. Science 1993;261:355–8.

12. Rawlings DJ, Saffran DC, Tsukada S, et al. Mutation of unique region of Bruton's tyrosine kinase in immunodeficient XID mice. Science 1993;261:358–61.

13. Khan WN, Alt FW, Gerstein RM, et al. Defective B cell development and function in Btk-deficient mice. Immunity 1995;3:283–99.

14. Kerner JD, Appleby MW, Mohr RN, et al. Impaired expansion of mouse B cell pro-genitors lacking Btk. Immunity 1995;3:301–12.

15. Anderson JS, Teutsch M, Dong Z, et al. An essential role for Bruton's [corrected] tyrosine kinase in the regulation of B-cell apoptosis. Proc Natl Acad Sci U S A 1996;93:10966–71.

16. de Weers M, Brouns GS, Hinshelwood S, et al. B-cell antigen receptor stimulation activates the human Bruton's tyrosine kinase, which is deficient in X-linked agam-maglobulinemia. J Biol Chem 1994;269:23857–60.

17. Aoki Y, Isselbacher KJ, Pillai S. Bruton tyrosine kinase is tyrosine phosphorylated and activated in pre-B lymphocytes and receptor-ligated B cells. Proc Natl Acad Sci U S A 1994;91:10606–9.

18. Takata M, Kurosaki T. A role for Bruton's tyrosine kinase in B cell antigen receptor-mediated activation of phospholipase C-gamma 2. J Exp Med 1996;184:31–40.

19. Irish JM, Czerwinski DK, Nolan GP, et al. Kinetics of B cell receptor signaling in human B cell subsets mapped by phosphospecific flow cytometry. J Immunol 2006;177:1581–9.

20. Egawa T, Albrecht B, Favier B, et al. Requirement for CARMA1 in antigen receptor-induced NF-kappa B activation and lymphocyte proliferation. Curr Biol 2003;13:1252–8.

21. Liu X, Zhan Z, Li D, et al. Intracellular MHC class II molecules promote TLR-triggered innate immune responses by maintaining activation of the kinase Btk. Nat Immunol 2011;12:416–24.

22. Gray P, Dunne A, Brikos C, et al. MyD88 adapter-like (Mal) is phosphorylated by Bruton's tyrosine kinase during TLR2 and TLR4 signal transduction. J Biol Chem 2006;281:10489–95.

23. de Gorter DJ, Beuling EA, Kersseboom R, et al. Bruton's tyrosine kinase and phospholipase Cgamma2 mediate chemokine-controlled B cell migration and homing. Immunity 2007;26:93–104.

24. de Weers M, Verschuren MC, Kraakman ME, et al. The Bruton's tyrosine kinase gene is expressed throughout B cell differentiation, from early precursor B cell stages preceding immunoglobulin gene rearrangement up to mature B cell stages. Eur J Immunol 1993;23:3109–14.

25. Mahajan S, Ghosh S, Sudbeck EA, et al. Rational design and synthesis of a novel anti-leukemic agent targeting Bruton's tyrosine kinase (BTK), LFM-A13 [alpha-cyano-beta-hydroxy-beta-methyl-N-(2, 5-dibromophenyl)propenamide]. J Biol Chem 1999;274:9587–99.

26. Honigberg LA, Smith AM, Sirisawad M, et al. The Bruton tyrosine kinase inhibitor PCI-32765 blocks B-cell activation and is efficacious in models of autoimmune disease and B-cell malignancy. Proc Natl Acad Sci U S A 2010;107:13075–80.

27. Davis RE, Ngo VN, Lenz G, et al. Chronic active B-cell-receptor signalling in diffuse large B-cell lymphoma. Nature 2010;463:88–92.

28. de Rooij MF, Kuil A, Kater AP, et al. Ibrutinib and idelalisib synergistically target BCR-controlled adhesion in MCL and CLL: a rationale for combination therapy. Blood 2015;125:2306–9.

29. de Rooij MF, Kuil A, Kraan W, et al. Ibrutinib and idelalisib target B cell receptor-but not CXCL12/CXCR4-controlled integrin-mediated adhesion in Waldenstrom macroglobulinemia. Haematologica 2016;101:e111–5.

30. Chen SS, Chang BY, Chang S, et al. BTK inhibition results in impaired CXCR4 chemokine receptor surface expression, signaling and function in chronic lymphocytic leukemia. Leukemia 2016;30:833–43.

31. Treon SP, Tripsas CK, Meid K, et al. Ibrutinib in previously treated Waldenstrom's macroglobulinemia. N Engl J Med 2015;372:1430–40.

32. Cao Y, Hunter ZR, Liu X, et al. The WHIM-like CXCR4(S338X) somatic mutation activates AKT and ERK, and promotes resistance to ibrutinib and other agents used in the treatment of Waldenstrom's Macroglobulinemia. Leukemia 2015;29:169–76.

33. Dubovsky JA, Beckwith KA, Natarajan G, et al. Ibrutinib is an irreversible molecular inhibitor of ITK driving a Th1-selective pressure in T lymphocytes. Blood 2013;122:2539–49.

34. Ping L, Ding N, Shi Y, et al. The Bruton's tyrosine kinase inhibitor ibrutinib exerts immunomodulatory effects through regulation of tumor-infiltrating macrophages. Oncotarget 2017;8:39218–29.

35. Treon SP, MK, Gustine J, et al. Long-term follow-up of previously treated patients who received ibrutinib for symptomatic Waldenstrom's Macroglobulinemia: update of pivotal clinical trial. Presented at the 59th ASH meeting. Atlanta, GA, 2017.

36. Gertz MA, Rue M, Blood E, et al. Multicenter phase 2 trial of rituximab for Waldenstrom macroglobulinemia (WM): an Eastern Cooperative Oncology Group Study (E3A98). Leuk Lymphoma 2004;45:2047–55.

37. Treon SP, Hunter ZR, Matous J, et al. Multicenter clinical trial of bortezomib in relapsed/refractory Waldenstrom's macroglobulinemia: results of WMCTG Trial 03-248. Clin Cancer Res 2007;13:3320–5.

38. Dimopoulos MA, Trotman J, Tedeschi A, et al. Ibrutinib for patients with rituximab-refractory Waldenstrom's macroglobulinaemia (iNNOVATE): an open-label substudy of an international, multicentre, phase 3 trial. Lancet Oncol 2017;18:241–50.

39. Treon SP, GJ, Meid K, et al. Ibrutinib is highly active as first line therapy in symptomatic Waldenstrom's Macroglobulinemia. Presented at the 59th ASH meeting. Atlanta, GA, 2017.

40. Yang G, LX, Chen J, et al. Targeting IRAK1/IRAK4 signaling in Waldenstrom's Macroglobulinemia. Presented at the 57th ASH meetting. Orlando, FL, 2015.

41. Woyach JA, Furman RR, Liu TM, et al. Resistance mechanisms for the Bruton's tyrosine kinase inhibitor ibrutinib. N Engl J Med 2014;370:2286–94.

42. Xu L, Tsakmaklis N, Yang G, et al. Acquired mutations associated with ibrutinib resistance in Waldenstrom macroglobulinemia. Blood 2017;129:2519–25.

43. Chen JG, LX, Chen J, et al. Acquisition of BTK C481S produces resistance to ibrutinib in MYD88 mutated WM and ABC DLBCL cells that is accompanied by ERK1/2 hyperactivation, and is targeted by the addition of the ERK1/2 inhibitor ulixertinib. Presented at the 58th ASH meeting. San Diego, CA, 2016.

44. Barakat FH, Medeiros LJ, Wei EX, et al. Residual monotypic plasma cells in patients with waldenstrom macroglobulinemia after therapy. Am J Clin Pathol 2011; 135:365–73.

45. Cao Y, Yang G, Hunter ZR, et al. The BCL2 antagonist ABT-199 triggers apoptosis, and augments ibrutinib and idelalisib mediated cytotoxicity in CXCR4 Wild-type and CXCR4 WHIM mutated Waldenstrom macroglobulinaemia cells. Br J Haematol 2015;170:134–8.

46. Davids MS, Roberts AW, Seymour JF, et al. Phase I first-in-human study of venetoclax in patients with relapsed or refractory Non-Hodgkin Lymphoma. J Clin Oncol 2017;35:826–33.

47. Caron F, Leong DP, Hillis C, et al. Current understanding of bleeding with ibrutinib use: a systematic review and meta-analysis. Blood Adv 2017;1:772–8.

48. Leong DP, Caron F, Hillis C, et al. The risk of atrial fibrillation with ibrutinib use: a systematic review and meta-analysis. Blood 2016;128:138–40.

49. Levade M, David E, Garcia C, et al. Ibrutinib treatment affects collagen and von Willebrand factor-dependent platelet functions. Blood 2014;124:3991–5.

50. Kamel S, Horton L, Ysebaert L, et al. Ibrutinib inhibits collagen-mediated but not ADP-mediated platelet aggregation. Leukemia 2015;29:783–7.

51. Bye AP, Unsworth AJ, Desborough MJ, et al. Severe platelet dysfunction in NHL patients receiving ibrutinib is absent in patients receiving acalabrutinib. Blood Adv 2017;1:2610–23.

52. McMullen JR, Boey EJ, Ooi JY, et al. Ibrutinib increases the risk of atrial fibrillation, potentially through inhibition of cardiac PI3K-Akt signaling. Blood 2014;124: 3829–30.

53. Li N, SZ, Liu Y, et al. BGB-3111 is a novel and highly selective Bruton's tyrosine kinase (BTK) inhibitor. Presented at the AACR 106th Annual Meeting. Philadelphia, PA, 2015.

54. Tam C, GA, Opat S, et al. The BTK inhibitor, Bgb-3111, is safe, tolerable, and highly active in patients with relapsed/refractory B-cell malignancies: initial report of a phase 1 first-in-human trial. Presented at the 57th ASH meeting. Orlando, FL, 2015.

55. Byrd JC, Furman RR, Coutre SE, et al. Targeting BTK with ibrutinib in relapsed chronic lymphocytic leukemia. N Engl J Med 2013;369:32–42.

56. Trotman J, OS, Marlton P, et al. Bruton's Tyrosine Kinase (BTK) Inhibitor BGB-3111 demonstrates high Very Good Partial Response (VGPR) rate in patients with Waldenstrom Macroglobuliemia (WM). Presented at the International Conference on Malignant Lymphoma biennial meeting Lugano. Switzerland, 2017.

57. Walter HS, Rule SA, Dyer MJ, et al. A phase 1 clinical trial of the selective BTK inhibitor ONO/GS-4059 in relapsed and refractory mature B-cell malignancies. Blood 2016;127:411–9.

58. Harrington BK, GM, Covey T, et al. ACP-196 is a second generation inhibitor of bruton tyrosine kinase (BTK) with enhanced target specificity. Presented at the 57th ASH annual meeting. Orlando, FL, 2015.

59. Byrd JC, Harrington B, O'Brien S, et al. Acalabrutinib (ACP-196) in relapsed chronic lymphocytic leukemia. N Engl J Med 2016;374:323–32.

60. Wang M, RS, Zinzani PL, et al. Efficacy and safety of acalabrutinib monotherapy in patients with relapsed/refractory mantle cell lymphoma in the phase 2 ACE-LY-004 study. Presented at the 59th ASH annual meeting. Atlanta, GA, 2017.

61. Ward R, NL, Arnold S, et al. A phase 1a study to investigate the safety, pharmacokinetics, and pharmacodynamics of the non covalent Bruton's Tyrosine Kinase inhibitor SNS-062 in healthy subjects:preliminary results. Presented at the 2nd International Conference on New Concepts in B-Cell Malignancies. Estoril, Portugal, 2016.

62. Neuman LL, WR, Arnold D, et al. First-in-human phase 1a study of the safety, pharmacokinetics, and pharmacodynamics of the noncovalent bruton tyrosine kinase (BTK) inhibitor SNS-062 in healthy subjects. Presented at the 58TH ASH annual meeting. San Diego, CA, 2016.

63. Castillo JJ, Gustine JN, Meid K, et al. Ibrutinib withdrawal symptoms in patients with Waldenstrom Macroglobulinemia. Haematologica 2018;103: e307–10.

64. Gustine JN, Meid K, Dubeau T, et al. Ibrutinib discontinuation in Waldenstrom macroglobulinemia: etiologies, outcomes, and IgM rebound. Am J Hematol 2018;93:511–7.

High-Dose Therapy and Hematopoietic Stem Cell Transplantation in Waldenström Macroglobulinemia

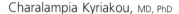

Charalampia Kyriakou, MD, PhD

KEYWORDS

- Transplantation • Waldenström macroglobulinemia • Autologous • Allogeneic

KEY POINTS

- Waldenström macroglobulinemia (WM) is an indolent low-grade non-Hodgkin lymphoma characterized by bone marrow infiltration by lymphoplasmacytic cells and associated clonal IgM paraproteinemia.
- Recent insights into the biology and genomic characteristics of WM have provided further platform for more targeted therapies. Despite the high response rates and better depth and duration of responses, however, the disease remains incurable.
- High-risk WM and patients not responding to conventional therapies have short survival.
- This review focuses on the use of the high-dose therapy with either autologous or allogeneic hematopoietic stem cell transplantation. Although transplantation could be associated with high treatment-related toxicity, it can salvage patients with WM failing other therapies.
- In the era of cellular immunotherapies, stem cell toxic therapies should be avoided at earlier treatment lines.

INTRODUCTION

Waldenström macroglobulinemia (WM)/lymphoplasmacytic lymphoma is a rare low-grade B cell lymphoma, characterized by bone marrow infiltration by lymphoplasmacytic cells and associated IgM monoclonal gammopathy.[1–3] The identification of recurrent mutations in the MYD88 and CXCR4 genes has significantly improved understanding of the disease biology.

The treatment approach of the disease, due to the diversity of clinical and biological features observed in WM patients, should be personalized, considering patient and disease factors, such as age, comorbidities, constitutional symptoms, cytopenias,

Department of Haematology, University College London, Huntley Street, London WC1E 6AG, UK
E-mail addresses: c.kyriakou@nhs.net; charalampia.kyriakou1@nhs.net

Hematol Oncol Clin N Am 32 (2018) 865–874
https://doi.org/10.1016/j.hoc.2018.05.013
0889-8588/18/Crown Copyright © 2018 Published by Elsevier Inc. All rights reserved.

IgM levels, presence of hyperviscosity, coagulopathy, cryoglobulinemia, cold agglutinin disease and peripheral neuropathy, need for rapid disease response, and candidacy for hematopoietic stem cell transplantation. WM patients with asymptomatic disease should be observed because survival similar to the general population has been reported.[4–6] Indications for treatment of symptomatic WM patients are based on symptoms and/or signs, as defined by international consensus panel recommendations. The advances on therapies for symptomatic WM patients at presentation or relapse using a variety of chemotherapeutic agents, alone or in combination, have improved disease response and outcomes. The International Prognostic Scoring System for WM (IPSSWM) has been validated as a reliable tool for treatment decision and it is important to use for the risk stratification for the treatment of WM patients.[7–10]

WM has no standard formally approved therapy and there is updated consensus treatment recommendations from a panel of experts, provided during the 7th International Workshop on WM.[11] Based on the available data and the experience in treating patients with low-grade lymphomas, treatment options for symptomatic WM disease include combinations of anti-CD20 monoclonal antibody with alkylating agents, steroids, proteasome inhibitors, purine analogs, and most recently B-cell receptor inhibitors. The combination of dexamethasone and anti-CD20 monoclonal antibody with cyclophosphamide, bendamustine, fludarabine, or proteasome inhibitors (rituximab) has been associated relatively low toxicity and achieved high and durable responses. The use of proteasome inhibitor can achieve rapid response and better control of hyperviscosity whereas chemotherapeutic drugs enable better nodal disease debulk.

For relapsed disease, the treatment options depend on the response and duration of response to previous line therapies, candidacy for transplantation, patient age, and overall condition. For patients who sustained response for greater than or equal to 24 months, administering the same regimen used as initial treatment could be considered. Otherwise, the use of alternate salvage single or combination treatments is also effective. Novel new agents offer further multiple options for subsequent relapses.

ROLE OF HIGH-DOSE THERAPY AND AUTOLOGOUS STEM CELL TRANSPLANTATION IN THE TREATMENT OF WALDENSTRÖM MACROGLOBULINEMIA

The role of high-dose therapy and autologous stem cell transplantation (ASCT) remains a controversial option, in the era of a new targeted highly effective drugs, for an indolent disease that frequently affects elderly patients.

For WM patients who are potential stem cell transplantation (SCT) candidates at first or subsequent relapses, it is important to avoid the use of stem cell toxic therapeutic agents for first-line therapy, to reduce the risk of compromising adequate stem cell mobilization. The use of purine analogs has been associated with stem cell harvest failure, and this was also reported in chronic lymphocytic leukemia and other low-grade lymphomas.[12,13] The 7th International Workshop on WM and updated National Comprehensive Cancer Network treatment recommendations specifically advise avoidance of purine nucleoside analogs for potential SCT candidates (**Box 1**).[11] Furthermore, the use of multiple therapy lines and disease responses after multiple relapses could be directly related to failure for hematopoietic stem cell harvest. The borderline patient age at presentation or at relapse and financial pressures are the reasons that stem cell harvest, cryopreservation, and storage have not been standard practice in most nations.

Information on SCT for WM was limited to small case series and retrospective reports (**Table 1**). In a small pilot study, 5 WM patients were treated as part of initial therapy with SCT using cyclophosphamide/granulocyte colony-stimulating factor for stem

---

Box 1
Primary or salvage treatment regimen for Waldenström macroglobulinemia by possible stem cell toxicity

Possible stem cell toxicity/and/or unknown
  Bendamustine ± rituximab
  Cladribine ± rituximab
  Chlorambucil
  Fludarabine ± rituximab
  Fludarabine/cyclophosphamide ± rituximab

Non–stem cell toxic regimens
  Alemtuzumab
  Bortezomib ± rituximab
  Bortezomib/dexamethasone
  Bortezomib/dexamethasone ± rituximab
  Cyclophosphamide/doxorubicin/vincristine/prednisolone/rituximab
  Carfizomib
  Everolimus
  Ibrutinib
  Ofatumumab
  Rituximab
  Rituximab/cyclophosphamide/dexamethasone

---

cell harvest and melphalan, 200 mg/m^2, as conditioning. At a median follow-up post-ASCT of 66 months (range, 56–75), all patients were evaluable, were alive without evidence of disease progression, and maintained a stable very good partial response (VGPR).[14]

Another group reported the outcome of ASCT on 6 WM patients. Two patients had the ASCT as first-line therapy and 4 after disease relapse. Melphalan was used as conditioning regimen, except in 1 patient who had addition of total body irradiation (TBI). The responses reported were high, with patients free of disease at 52 months, 15 months, 12 months, and 2 months post-ASCT.[15]

Eight WM patients, in another study, underwent melphalan-based regimen and ASCT; 7 achieved partial response, 1 achieved complete response, and 5 were alive and relapse-free at 6 to 77 months after ASCT.[16]

A prospective study of high-dose therapy and SCT as part of first-line treatment of indolent lymphomas, reported by the German Indolent Lymphoma Working Group, included 12 patients with WM. After an optional cytoreduction with alkylators or fludarabine, patients received salvage with dexa-mini-BEAM (Carmustine, Etoposide,

---

Table 1
Autologous stem cell transplantation in Waldenström macroglobulinemia

Author, Year	N	Median Follow-Up (mo)	Progression-free Survival	Overall Survival
Dreger & Schmitz,[17] 2007	12	69	Median PFS: 69 mo	100% at 69 mo
Caravita et al,[14] 2009	5	66	100% at 66 mo	—
Anagnostopoulos et al,[20] 2006	10	63	65% at 3 y	70% at 3 y
Gilleece et al,[18] 2008	9	44	Disease-free survival: 43% at 4 y	73% at 4 y
Kyriakou, 2010[22,31]	158	50	40% at 5 y	69% at 5 y

Cytarabine, Melphalan) for stem cell mobilization and remission induction followed by myeloablative therapy with TBI in combination with high-dose cyclophosphamide and SCT. All patients achieved VGPR and 6 patients had disease progression at a median time of 69 months and with median time to retreatment of 82 months.[17]

The British Society of Blood and Marrow Transplantation reported 9 patients with lymphoplasmacytic lymphoma who were treated at subsequent relapses with ASCT. The median follow-up was 44 months, with a 4-year progression-free survival (PFS) of 43% and an overall survival (OS) at 4 years of 73%.[18]

In another study on 24 heavily pretreated WM patients who received ASCT with either melphalan or cyclophosphamide-based conditioning and 9 of them with additional TBI, the results showed responses in 23 of 24 patients, and 9 of 23 evaluable patients achieved a complete response.[19]

A retrospective review from the Center for International Blood and Marrow Transplant Research (CIBMTR) database reported the ASCT outcomes on 9 WM patients with relapse or refractory disease and 1 patient treated as part of first-line therapy. The reported PFS and OS at 3 years were 65% and 70%, respectively, with a median follow-up of 63 months.[20]

Tournilhac and colleagues reported the experience on ASCT on 19 WM patients in 2003. The median time from WM diagnosis to transplant was 36 months. The response rate post ASCT was 95%. Within a median follow-up of 18 months, 12 patients were alive at 10 months to 81 months and 8 patients were relapse-free at 10 months to 34 months.[21]

The French group updated their experience on ASCT on 32 heavily pretreated WM patients. The conditioning regimen was with BEAM regimen in 13 patients, TBI/melphalan in 9 patients, and TBI/cyclophosphamide in 7 patients, and the median follow-up was 45 months. The median event-free survival was 32 months, the 5-year survival was 58%, and the transplant-related mortality was 12.5%. Thus, ASCT can achieve long-term responses even in heavily pretreated patients.

The European Society for Blood and Marrow Transplantation (EBMT) Registry published outcomes on 158 WM patients transplanted between 1991 and 2005. The median age at ASCT was 53 years, and at presentation 37% of the patients had intermediate-risk disease and 54% had a high-risk disease as defined by the IPSSWM; 21% of the WM patients were autografted in first VGPR (VGPR1), 9% in second VGPR (VGPR2), and 5% in the third or later VGPR (VGPR3); 31% of the patients were autografted in first partial response (PR1) and 19% in the second or later partial response (PR2). Granulocyte colony-stimulating factor alone or in combination with chemotherapy in 77% were used for stem cell mobilization. Conditioning regimen was chemotherapy-based in most of the patients and the median follow-up was 4.2 years. Complete remission (CR) was reported in 22%, VGPR in 50%, partial response in 15%, and 11% had disease relapse or progression; 68% of the patients were alive; and 32% died, with 26% dying of disease progression. Incidence of non-relapse mortality (NRM) was 3.8% at 1 year, 4.6% at 3 years, and 5.6% at 5 years post-ASCT. This study reported cumulative incidence of secondary malignancies after ASCT of 8.4% at 5 years. In addition, the analysis stressed that the prior use of fludarabine was found an independent factor for secondary malignancies and was associated with harvest failure and need for further mobilization attempts. The OS rate at 5 years was 69% and 49% patients were alive and remained progression-free, with estimated PFS rates of 40% at 5 years; 45% relapsed or progressed within a median time from transplantation of 1.3 years and the estimated relapse rate (RR) was 48% at 5 years, respectively. Chemorefractory disease greater than or equal to 3 prior therapy lines and poor performance were unfavorable factors for NRM, RR, PFS, and OS. A subgroup analysis was performed on 69 patients autografted after a first response (VGPR1/PR1) and the estimated PFS at 5 years was 52% and OS at 5 years was 77%.[22]

At the 56th ASH meeting, the EBMT presented the updated European experience on 615 WM patients treated with ASCT. The median time from diagnosis to transplant was 19 months and the median follow-up was 53 months. The disease status at ASCT was PR1, VGPR1, or 1st complete remission (CR1) in 325 patients, whereas 176 patients were autografted in second, third, or later response; and 47 patients (4%) had primary refractory or progressive disease at ASCT. The reported NRM, RR, PFS, and OS at 5 years were, 7%, 47%, 46%, and 65%, respectively. Relapse incidence was significantly lower when ASCT was performed in first maximum disease response (CR1, PR1, and VGPR1) compared with when the ASCT was used in subsequent complete or partial responses or with refractory disease (39% vs 53%; $P = .001$), translating into a significant disease-free survival (50% vs 40%, $P = .004$) and OS benefit (71% vs 63%; $P = .033$) for the patients transplanted early.[23]

DISCUSSION

Although the published data are from small series and retrospective studies, all suggested that ASCT is a feasible treatment option for WM and produces durable responses with acceptable ASCT-related toxicity. The international WM and the EBMT consensus recommendations suggest that ASCT should not be offered as first-line therapy but should be considered a salvage treatment option for transplant-eligible patients at first or subsequent disease relapses. The consensus is for the ASCT candidates to avoid first-line therapies with stem cell toxic chemotherapeutic combinations (see **Box 1**). In the era of major advances in novel agent development, ASCT could also be a bridging therapy with lasting responses. It is an effective treatment option for transplant-eligible patients but should be offered at early relapses that can result in higher, deeper, and lasting response rates with relatively low toxicity. ASCT was not found to be beneficial for patients who were transplanted with chemorefractory disease or those who were exposed to more than 3 lines of therapy. These refractory patients should not proceed to ASCT and should be considered for clinical trials.

ROLE FOR HIGH-DOSE THERAPY AND ALLOGENEIC STEM CELL TRANSPLANTATION IN THE TREATMENT OF WALDENSTRÖM MACROGLOBULINEMIA

The place of high-dose therapy and allogeneic stem cell transplantation (alloSCT) in the treatment algorithm of the WM and other indolent lymphomas is gradually becoming more challenging and remains controversial. No prospective studies were performed and the published data on the role of alloSCT for patients with WM are limited and from retrospective reports. The older age of patients at diagnosis, the increasing new targeted therapeutic options for the WM patients, and the difficulty to identify those patients destined to do poorly at diagnosis all may have contributed to the limited use of alloSCT and outcome data. The unacceptably high NRM reported after myeloablative conditioning (MAC) alloSCT also played a significant role.[20,21] NRM after alloSCT has decreased in virtually all lymphoma subtypes over the past decade. This has largely been attributed to the introduction of reduced-intensity conditioning (RIC). The RIC protocols were designed to reduce NRM but to preserve the clinically important graft-versus-lymphoma effect that has been reported in other subtypes of lymphomas. The initial data on the use of alloSCT for WM are mainly from case reports on WM patients with refractory or multiply relapsed WM.

A retrospective review on 5 WM patients treated with MAC alloSCT, using busulfan/cyclophosphamide conditioning, reported that, with a median follow-up of 32 months, 4 of the 5 patients were alive and disease-free. In addition, a further gradual drop of the serum IgM levels was observed in all patients, suggesting an active graft-versus-WM effect.[24]

An earlier case report on a 62-year-old man with refractory WM who underwent an RIC alloSCT[25] and small case series on 3 WM patients reported encouraging outcomes by Anagnostopoulos and colleagues.[26] In another case report, a 52-year-old patient received RIC alloSCT for primary refractory WM disease but without adequate clinical response. The patient received donor lymphocyte infusion (DLI) for mixed chimerism and primary refractory disease and converted to full donor chimerism. The DLI was complicated with limited controlled chronic graft-versus-host disease (GVHD) but the WM disease response was escalated from primary refractory to complete remission suggesting also graft-versus-WM effect.[27]

Another systematic review of 6 heavily pretreated WM patients having alloSCT reported prolong survival in 3 of the 6 patients. Two patients died from NRM and 1 from progressive disease.[28]

Tournilhac and colleagues[21] reported results on 10 WM patients with relapsed refractory disease, treated with MAC alloSCT. Six patients were alive at 3 months, 23 months, 50 months, 59 months, 74 months, and 76 months; however, the NRM was high at 40%.

Tournilhac and colleagues[21] presented at the Interntional Workshop on WM in 2003 a retrospective review of 22 WM patients, 11 treated with RIC and 11 patients with MAC alloSCT. The NRM was 27%, the median event-free survival had not been reached; the OS was 68% at 5 years for the RIC group. For the patients treated with MAC alloSCT, the NRM was 36%, the median survival was 36 months, and OS at 5 years was 54%.

The CIBMTR registry analysis reported the outcomes on 26 WM patients treated with alloSCT. MAC alloSCT was used in 58% of this group and, after a median follow-up of 65 months, 35% of all patients were alive. NRM was 40%, and estimated PFS and OS at 3 years were 31% and 46%, respectively.[20]

Meniane and colleagues[27] reviewed reports on 46 WM patients receiving alloSCT. MAC regimen was used in 34 and RIC in 12 patients. Survival rates were 46% and NRM 40% at 3 years.

Gilleece and colleagues reported the experience on allo SCT in 7 WM patients treated with RIC and 2 with MAC. The median follow-up was 32 months, the NRM at 1 year was 44%, and the PFS and OS at 4 years were 44% and 56%, respectively.[18]

Although the data from these initial reports were from small patient series, all reported promising outcomes on mainly heavily pretreated or refractory to treatment WM patients. All reports pointed to a high transplant-related toxicity, but they also suggested that, the alloSCT rescued and prolonged the survival in a high-risk group of WM patients, suggesting that alloSCT is feasible in a population of eligible WM patients.

Garnier and colleagues[29] updated the French experience and reported outcomes of alloSCT on 25 WM patients 13 treated with MAC and 11 with RIC alloSCT; 44% had primary refractory disease and a median of 3 prior therapy lines at the time of alloSCT. The median follow-up was 64 months among survivors and the reported overall response rate was 92%, with 50% of the evaluable patients obtaining complete response. The 5-year PFS and OS were 58% and 67%, respectively. This retrospective report showed alloSCTs yielded a high rate of complete responses and were potentially curative in a refractory, poor prognosis group of WM patients.

At the 5th International Workshop on WM in 2008, Maloney and colleagues[30] presented, data on 13 WM patients with advanced stage, refractory disease, heavily pretreated patients who underwent allograft with low-dose TBI (2 Gy) and fludarabine. The response rate was 91%, the NRM was 31%, and the 4-year PFS and OS rates were 60%. Longer survival was observed in those patients who developed extensive chronic GVHD, suggesting the existence of a graft-versus-WM effect.

The EBMT Lymphoma Working Party reported the experience on 86 WM from the EBMT Registry; 37 patients were treated with MAC and 49 with RIC alloSCT; and 8 patients had failed a previous ASCT and 69% had chemosensitive disease at the time of alloSCT. The median follow-up of survivors was 50 months and the overall response rate was 75.6%. The NRM at 3 years was 33% for the MAC and 23% for the RIC patients. The 3-year relapse rate was 11% for the MAC transplants and 25% for the RIC. The 5-year PFS and OS were 56% and 62%, respectively, for the MAC group, and 49% and 64% for the RIC, respectively. Chronic GVHD was associated with higher NRM and a lower relapse rate, leading to the improved PFS. This report showed that alloSCT can induce durable remissions in heavily pretreated WM patients. The low relapse rate in patients developing chronic GVHD suggests the existence of a clinically relevant graft-versus-WM effect (**Table 2**).[31]

The EBMT reported at the 58th ASH meeting the long-term outcome of alloSCT on 260 WM patients transplanted between 2001 and 2013. RIC was the conditioning used for 66% of the patients. After a median follow-up for living patients of 57 months, the 5-year NRM, IR, PFS, and OS were 29%, 24%, 47% and 55%, respectively. Univariate and multivariate analyses to identify risk factors for alloSCT outcomes identified, the performance status for NRM, the disease status for RR, and performance status and MAC for OS as significant predictors of an adverse outcome after multivariable adjustment. Although RIC patients tended to have a lower NRM and a better PFS than MAC patients, this was not statistically significant, suggesting that RIC patients had a better survival after relapse; 45 patients were treated with DLI and results showed 60% response, which was complete in 55% supporting the data from other reports of graft-versus-WM effect.[32]

The CIBMTR published the outcomes of alloSCT on 144 WM patients transplanted between 2001 and 2013. MAC was used in 50% of the patients and RIC in the other 50%. Disease status at the time of alloSCT was chemosensitive for 57% and progressive disease in 22%, and 13% failed a previous ASCT. The NRM, RR, PFS, and OS rates for all patients at 5 years were 30%, 24%, 46%, and 52%, respectively. Patients with chemosensitive disease and better pretransplant disease status experienced significantly superior OS. The intensity of the conditioning did not have a insignificant impact on OS, PFS,

Table 2
Allogeneic stem cell transplantation in Waldenström macroglobulinemia

Author, Year	N	Follow-up (Median)	Nonrelapse Mortality	Progression-Free Survival	Overall Survival
Anagnostopoulos et al,[20] 2006	MAC: 21 RIC: 5	75 mo	40% at 3 y	31% at 3 y	46% at 3 y
Garnier et al,[29] 2010	MAC: 12 RIC: 13	63 mo	25% at 1 y	58% at 5 y	67% at 5 y
Kyriakou, 2010	MAC: 37 RIC: 49	63 mo 44 mo	33% at 3 y 23% at 3 y	56% at 5 y 49% at 5 y	62% at 5 y 64% at 5 y
Cornell et al,[33] 2017	MAC: 67	70 mo	12% and 24% at 1 y and 5 y	69% and 50% at 1 y and 5 y	73% and 55% at 1 y and 5 y
	RIC: 67	70 mo	15% and 39% at 1 y and 5 y	68% and 41% at 1 y and 5 y	73% and 45% at 1 y and 5 y

NRM, and RR outcomes.[33] At 5 years, the rates for the NRM for MAC/RIC were 24%/39%, the RRs were 27%/21%, the PFSs were 50%/41%, and the OS rates were 55%/45%, respectively. The most common causes of death reported were primary disease and GVHD. AlloSCT yielded durable survival in select WM patients with WM.

DISCUSSION

Although there are major diagnostic and therapeutic advances in the management of WM patients, the disease remains incurable with the current available therapies. After multiple relapses, the duration of response shortens and ultimately the disease becomes refractory. There is also a recognized group of patients with poor prognosis disease per the IPSSWM. The international consensus recommendations suggest that alloSCT should be ideally undertaken in the context of a clinical trial. Due to the rarity of the disease, older group of patients, and smaller subgroup of WM patients that might need the alloSCT approach, clinical trials evaluating alloSCT in WM are challenging if not impossible.

The information from the published data from the small series and retrospective studies suggest that a group of young alloSCT eligible WM patients can be still rescued. The even most important message from these studies was that alloSCT could salvage even patients transplanted after multiple prior line therapies or those patients who had primary chemorefractory disease at the time of transplantation. Furthermore, despite the heavily pretreated patient population, the responses were lasting, although at higher rates of treatment related toxicity. To reduce toxicity, the RIC has become the choice of alloSCT in an elderly group of lymphoma patients.

The association of chronic GVHD with better PFS and lower relapse rates, together with the fact that DLI for persistent or relapse disease could escalate disease responses to durable remissions, favors the existence of graft-versus-WM effect. GVHD could add to toxicity but these patients who survived the toxicity of alloSCT can achieve long-lasting progression-free remissions from this approach.[31,33]

The transplant treatment option should remain a possible therapy at advanced stage, unless patients belong to the primary refractory to conventional therapies group, and then the overall short-term and long-term benefits to these patients should be considered and the procedure proceeded at earlier stage. AlloSCT should remain an option for WM patients who experience failure of other therapies, including ASCT.

Both autologous and allogeneic transplants are used in other types of low-grade/indolent lymphomas for relapse disease. The critical decision in the era of new targeted therapies is identifying the group of patients who will have the benefit and the timing of the transplant, so high treatment-related toxicity and, in cases of autologous transplant, chemoimmunotherapy or new-agent therapy resistance can be avoided. The coordinated use of the new drugs could be incorporated as a bridge to SCT or post-SCT to reduce further disease relapse in a selected transplant-eligible group of WM patients, and this approach could broaden therapeutic options especially in high-risk patients.

REFERENCES

1. Harris NL, Jaffe ES, Diebold J, et al. World Health Organization classification of neoplastic diseases of the hematopoietic and lymphoid tissues: report of the Clinical Advisory Committee meeting-Airlie House, Virginia, November 1997. J Clin Oncol 1999;17(12):3835–49.
2. Swerdlow SH, International Agency for Research on Cancer, World Health Organization. WHO classification of tumours of haematopoietic and lymphoid tissues. 4th edition. Lyon (France): International Agency for Research on Cancer; 2008.

3. Swerdlow SH, Kuzu I, Dogan A, et al. The many faces of small B cell lymphomas with plasmacytic differentiation and the contribution of MYD88 testing. Virchows Arch 2016;468(3):259–75.
4. Phekoo KJ, Jack RH, Davies E, et al, South Thames Haematology Specialist Committee. The incidence and survival of Waldenström's Macroglobulinaemia in South East England. Leuk Res 2008;32(1):55–9.
5. Garcia-Sanz R, Montoto S, Torrequebrada A, et al. Waldenström macroglobulinaemia: presenting features and outcome in a series with 217 cases. Br J Haematol 2001;115(3):575–82.
6. Baldini L, Goldaniga M, Guffanti A, et al. Immunoglobulin M monoclonal gammopathies of undetermined significance and indolent Waldenström's macroglobulinemia recognize the same determinants of evolution into symptomatic lymphoid disorders: proposal for a common prognostic scoring system. J Clin Oncol 2005;23(21):4662–8.
7. Morel P, Duhamel A, Gobbi P, et al. International prognostic scoring system for Waldenström macroglobulinemia. Blood 2009;113(18):4163–70.
8. Morel P, Merlini G. Can ISSWM be used for making treatment decisions? Clin Lymphoma Myeloma Leuk 2011;11(1):121–3.
9. Morel P, Merlini G. Risk stratification in Waldenström macroglobulinemia. Expert Rev Hematol 2012;5(2):187–99.
10. Morel P, Monconduit M, Jacomy D, et al. patients with the description of a new scoring system and its validation on 253 other patients. Blood 2000;96(3):852–8.
11. Dimopoulos MA, Kastritis E, Owen RG, et al. Treatment recommendations for patients with Waldenström macroglobulinemia (WM) and related disorders: IWWM-7 consensus. Blood 2014;124(9):1404–11.
12. Nichols GL, Skerrett DL. Peripheral blood stem cell mobilization and harvesting after fludarabine therapy for low-grade lymphoma and chronic lymphocytic leukemia. Stem Cells Dev 2005;14(1):3–5.
13. Gribben JG. Stem cell transplantation in chronic lymphocytic leukemia. Biol Blood Marrow Transplant 2009;15(1 Suppl):53–8.
14. Caravita T, Siniscalchi A, Tendas A, et al. High-dose therapy with autologous PBSC transplantation in the front-line treatment of Waldenström's macroglobulinemia. Bone Marrow Transplant 2009;43(7):587–8.
15. Desikan R, Dhodapkar M, Siegel D, et al. High-dose therapy with autologous haemopoietic stem cell support for Waldenström's macroglobulinaemia. Br J Haematol 1999;105(4):993–6.
16. Munshi NC, Barlogie B. Role for high-dose therapy with autologous hematopoietic stem cell support in Waldenström's macroglobulinemia. Semin Oncol 2003;30(2):282–5.
17. Dreger P, Schmitz N. Autologous stem cell transplantation as part of first-line treatment of Waldenström's macroglobulinemia. Biol Blood Marrow Transplant 2007;13(5):623–4.
18. Gilleece MH, Pearce R, Linch DC, et al. The outcome of haemopoietic stem cell transplantation in the treatment of lymphoplasmacytic lymphoma in the UK: a British Society Bone Marrow Transplantation study. Hematology 2008;13(2):119–27.
19. Anagnostopoulos A, Giralt S. Stem cell transplantation (SCT) for Waldenström's macroglobulinemia (WM). Bone Marrow Transplant 2002;29(12):943–7.
20. Anagnostopoulos A, Hari PN, Perez WS, et al. Autologous or allogeneic stem cell transplantation in patients with Waldenström's macroglobulinemia. Biol Blood Marrow Transplant 2006;12(8):845–54.

21. Tournilhac O, Leblond V, Tabrizi R, et al. Transplantation in Waldenström's macroglobulinemia—the French experience. Semin Oncol 2003;30(2):291–6.
22. Kyriakou C, Canals C, Sibon D, et al. High-dose therapy and autologous stem-cell transplantation in Waldenström macroglobulinemia: the Lymphoma Working Party of the European Group for Blood and Marrow Transplantation. J Clin Oncol 2010;28(13):2227–32.
23. Kyriakou C. Autologous Stem Cell Transplantation (ASCT) for the Treatment of Patients with Waldenström's Macroglobulinemia/Lymphoplasmacytic Lymphoma (WM/LPL). a Risk Factor Analysis By the European Society for Blood and Marrow Transplantation (EBMT) Lymphoma Working Party. 56 th Annual American Society of Hematology Meeting. San Francisco, December 1–4, 2014.
24. Stakiw J, Kim DH, Kuruvilla J, et al. Evidence of graft-versus-Waldenström's macroglobulinaemia effect after allogeneic stem cell transplantation: a single centre experience. Bone Marrow Transplant 2007;40(4):369–72.
25. Ueda T, Hatanaka K, Kosugi S, et al. Successful non-myeloablative allogeneic peripheral blood stem cell transplantation (PBSCT) for Waldenström's macroglobulinemia with severe pancytopenia. Bone Marrow Transplant 2001;28(6):609–11.
26. Anagnostopoulos A, Dimopoulos MA, Aleman A, et al. High-dose chemotherapy followed by stem cell transplantation in patients with resistant Waldenström's macroglobulinemia. Bone Marrow Transplant 2001;27(10):1027–9.
27. Meniane JC, El-Cheikh J, Faucher C, et al. Long-term graft-versus-Waldenström macroglobulinemia effect following reduced intensity conditioning allogeneic stem cell transplantation. Bone Marrow Transplant 2007;40(2):175–7.
28. Anagnostopoulos A, Aleman A, Giralt S. Autologous and allogeneic stem cell transplantation in Waldenström's macroglobulinemia: review of the literature and future directions. Semin Oncol 2003;30(2):286–90.
29. Garnier A, Robin M, Larosa F, et al. Allogeneic hematopoietic stem cell transplantation allows long-term complete remission and curability in high-risk Waldenström's macroglobulinemia. Results of a retrospective analysis of the Societe Francaise de Greffe de Moelle et de Therapie Cellulaire. Haematologica 2010; 95(6):950–5.
30. Maloney DG, Anderson LD. Evidence for GVWM following mini-allo in WM. Fred Hutchinson Cancer Research Center (FHCRC) and the University of Washington, Seattle, WA, USA. Abstract 147; Session VIII: Transplant Therapy of Waldenström's Macroglobulinemia; International Waldenstrom Macroglobulinemia Workshop; Stockholm, Sweden, 2008.
31. Kyriakou C, Canals C, Cornelissen JJ, et al. Allogeneic stem-cell transplantation in patients with Waldenström macroglobulinemia: report from the Lymphoma Working Party of the European Group for Blood and Marrow Transplantation. J Clin Oncol 2010;28(33):4926–34.
32. Kyriakou C. Long-Term Outcome of Allogeneic Stem Cell Transplantation (allo-SCT) in Patients with Waldenström Macroglobulinemia (WM)-a Retrospective Study of the Lymphoma Working Party of the European Society for Blood and Marrow Transplantation (EBMT) 58th Annual American Society of Hematology Meeting. San Diego, December, 2016.
33. Cornell RF, Bachanova V, D'Souza A, et al. Allogeneic transplantation for relapsed Waldenström macroglobulinemia and lymphoplasmacytic lymphoma. Biol Blood Marrow Transplant 2017;23(1):60–6.

Novel Approaches in Waldenström Macroglobulinemia

Michael A. Spinner, MD[a,1], Gaurav Varma, MD, MSPH[b,1],
Ranjana H. Advani, MD[a,]*

KEYWORDS

- Waldenström macroglobulinemia • PI3K • mTOR • Akt • Syk • CXCR4 • BCL-2
- XPO1

KEY POINTS

- Recent advances in the understanding of Waldenström macroglobulinemia (WM) biology have led to a plethora of novel therapeutic strategies.
- The success of ibrutinib in WM has shifted treatment paradigms away from conventional chemoimmunotherapy approaches.
- Recognition of high-risk genomic subgroups as well as mechanisms of acquired resistance to ibrutinib have led to targeting of additional pathways.
- In this article, the authors review ongoing and emerging trials of novel therapies in WM that target the B-cell receptor pathway beyond ibrutinib, toll-like receptor pathway, chemokine signaling, apoptotic pathway, chromatin remodeling, protein transport, the immune microenvironment, and CD19-directed immunotherapy.

INTRODUCTION

Historically, treatment strategies for Waldenström macroglobulinemia (WM) have been extrapolated from low-grade lymphoma and multiple myeloma (MM). Recent advances in the understanding of the genomic landscape of WM, intracellular B-cell signaling pathways, cytokine signaling, and the immune microenvironment have created an opportunity for the rational development of novel therapeutic strategies

Disclosure Statement: Dr R.H. Advani has received institutional research support from Pharmacyclics, Genentech, and Bristol-Myers Squibb, and honoraria for advisory board participation from Bayer, Pharmacyclics, AstraZeneca, Genentech, and Gilead. The other authors declare no relevant conflicts of interest.
[a] Division of Oncology, Department of Medicine, Stanford University, Stanford Cancer Institute, 875 Blake Wilbur Drive, Stanford, CA 94305, USA; [b] Department of Medicine, NewYork-Presbyterian Hospital/Weill Cornell Medicine, 525 East 68th Street, New York, NY
[1] Contributed equally.
* Corresponding author.
E-mail address: radvani@stanford.edu

(Fig. 1). Genetic studies from patients with WM have identified recurrent somatic mutations in *MYD88* in greater than 90% of patients as well as mutations of *CXCR4* in 30% to 40% of patients.[1,2] The latter significantly affects the depth of response to ibrutinib, a Bruton's tyrosine kinase (BTK) inhibitor recently approved by the US Food and Drug Administration (FDA) specifically for WM.[3] Additional mutations in various genes involved in the B-cell receptor (BCR) pathway, toll-like receptor (TLR) signaling, CXCR4 signaling, apoptotic pathway, and chromatin remodeling have also been identified in WM.[2] In this article, the authors review ongoing and emerging trials with novel therapies for patients with WM (**Tables 1** and **2**). Other established therapies, including alkylating agents, monoclonal antibodies, proteasome inhibitors, BTK inhibitors, and stem cell transplantation, are reviewed in additional articles.

TARGETING THE B-CELL RECEPTOR PATHWAY BEYOND BRUTON'S TYROSINE KINASE

Aberrant signaling through the BCR pathway has been implicated in the development of many B-cell malignancies, including WM.[4] The success of ibrutinib validated blockade of the BCR pathway as a viable strategy for WM. BCR signaling also involves several proteins upstream of BTK, including spleen tyrosine kinase (Syk) and the various components of the phosphatidylinositol-4,5-bisphosphate 3-kinase/Akt/

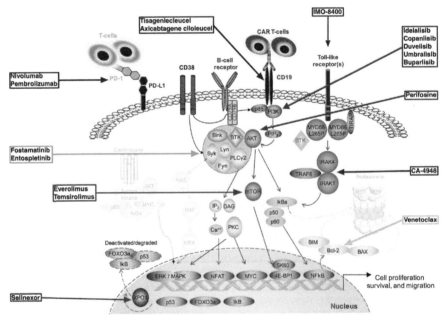

Fig. 1. Novel and established therapeutic targets in WM. Numerous novel agents are in preclinical and clinical development for molecular targets involved in WM cell survival. These include drugs that target BCR signaling (*green*), various protein kinases and adaptor proteins of the PI3K/Akt/mTOR pathway (*red*), and the TLR pathway (*purple*). Additional novel agents target proteins involved in the apoptotic pathway, such as BCL-2 (*yellow*), or protein transport such as XPO1 (*gray*). Finally, extracellular proteins like PD-L1 and CD19 (*blue*) represent promising targets for powerful new immunotherapies. (*Adapted from* Paulus A, Ailawadhi S, Chanan-Khan A. Novel therapeutic targets in Waldenstrom macroglobulinemia. Best Pract Res Clin Haematol 2016;29(2):218; with permission.)

Table 1
Completed trials of novel agents for relapsed or refractory Waldenström macroglobulinemia

Novel Agent	Molecular Target	Phase	Study Population	N	ORR in WM	Reference
Entospletinib	BCR signaling	Phase 2	R/R WM	17	24% (6% PR, 18% MR)	Assouline et al,[14] 2017
Idelalisib	BCR signaling	Phase 1	R/R indolent NHL	9	56% (11% PR, 45% MR)	Coutre et al,[15] 2015
Idelalisib	BCR signaling	Phase 2	R/R indolent NHL	10	80% (70% PR, 10% MR)	Gopal et al,[16] 2014
Idelalisib + entospletinib	BCR signaling	Phase 2	R/R indolent NHL	2	50% (50% PR)	Barr et al,[18] 2016
Copanlisib	BCR signaling	Phase 2	R/R indolent NHL	6	25% (25% PR)	Dreyling et al,[19] 2017
Duvelisib	BCR signaling	Phase 1	R/R indolent NHL	4	25% (25% MR)	Flinn et al,[20] 2018
Perifosine	BCR signaling	Phase 2	R/R WM	37	38% (8% PR, 30% MR)	Ghobrial et al,[24] 2010
Everolimus	BCR signaling	Phase 2	R/R WM	60	73% (50% PR, 23% MR)	Ghobrial et al,[25] 2014
Everolimus + bortezomib + rituximab	BCR signaling	Phase 1/2	R/R WM	46	87% (4% CR, 46% PR, 37% MR)	Ghobrial et al,[26] 2015
Temsirolimus	BCR signaling	Phase 2	R/R indolent NHL	3	33% (33% MR)	Smith et al,[27] 2010
Sapanisertib	BCR signaling	Phase 1	R/R MM or NHL	4	50% (25% PR, 25% MR)	Ghobrial et al,[28] 2016
Venetoclax	Apoptotic pathway	Phase 1	R/R NHL	4	100% (100% PR)	Davids et al,[48] 2017
Panobinostat	Chromatin remodeling	Phase 2	R/R WM	38	48% (17% PR, 31% MR)	Ghobrial et al,[57] 2011
Pembrolizumab	Immune microenvironment	Phase 2	R/R indolent NHL	3	33% (33% MR)	Ding et al,[68] 2017

Abbreviations: N, number of patients with Waldenström macroglobulinemia; R/R, relapsed or refractory.

Table 2
Ongoing trials of novel agents for Waldenström macroglobulinemia

Novel Agent	Molecular Target of Novel Agent	Phase	Study Population	Trial Number
Idelalisib + obinutuzumab	BCR signaling	Phase 2	R/R WM	NCT02962401
Idelalisib + tirabrutinib + obinurtuzumab	BCR signaling	Phase 1b	R/R CLL or NHL[a]	NCT02457598
Idelalisib + pembrolizumab	BCR signaling	Phase 2	R/R CLL or indolent NHL[a]	NCT02332980
Copanlisib	BCR signaling	Phase 3	R/R indolent NHL[a]	NCT02369016
Copanlisib + rituximab	BCR signaling	Phase 3	R/R indolent NHL[a]	NCT02367040
BR/RCHOP ± copanlisib	BCR signaling	Phase 3	R/R indolent NHL[a]	NCT02626455
Buparlisib + rituximab	BCR signaling	Phase 1	R/R indolent NHL[a]	NCT02049541
Umbralisib	BCR signaling	Phase 2	R/R indolent NHL[a]	NCT03364231
CA-4948 (IRAK4/1)	TLR pathway	Phase 1	R/R NHL[a]	NCT03328078
Ulocuplumab + ibrutinib	Chemokine signaling BCR signaling	Phase 1/2	WM with CXCR4 mutations	NCT03225716
Venetoclax	Apoptotic pathway	Phase 2	R/R WM	NCT02677324
Panobinostat + everolimus	Chromatin remodeling BCR signaling	Phase 1/2	R/R MM or NHL[a]	NCT00918333
Pembrolizumab + ibrutinib	Immune microenvironment BCR signaling	Phase 1	R/R NHL[a]	NCT02950220
Nivolumab + lenalidomide	Immune microenvironment	Phase 1/2	R/R HL or NHL[a]	NCT03015896
CD19–28z CAR T cells	CD19-directed immunotherapy	Phase 1/2	R/R indolent NHL[a]	NCT00466531

Abbreviations: BR, bendamustine/rituximab; HL, Hodgkin lymphoma; NCT, National Clinical Trial; RCHOP, rituximab, cyclophosphamide, doxorubicin, vincristine, prednisone.
[a] Includes patients with WM.

mammalian target of rapamycin (PI3K/Akt/mTOR) pathway, providing several rational drug targets.

Syk is involved in initiation and amplification of the BCR signal.[5] In malignant B cells, Syk interacts with PI3K to phosphorylate BTK leading to activation of phospholipase Cγ and increased NF-kB signaling as well as providing parallel signaling through Akt/mTOR.[6,7] Both Syk and the PI3K/Akt/mTOR axis are dysregulated in many B-cell malignancies, including WM.[8] Syk inhibition has been shown to induce apoptosis in B-cell lymphoma cell lines and primary tumors. Similar studies conducted in WM cell lines demonstrate that mutated MYD88[L265P] activates the PI3K/Akt/mTOR axis with decreased expression of PTEN along with expected increases in phosphorylated-Akt, phosphorylated-mTOR, rapamycin-sensitive mTOR complex 1 (mTORC1), and rapamycin-resistant mTOR complex 2 (mTORC2). These findings provide a rationale for targeting Syk and the PI3K/Akt/mTOR axis in patients with WM.[1,9–11]

Spleen Tyrosine Kinase Inhibitors

Two oral Syk inhibitors, fostamatinib and entospletinib, have been studied in preclinical models and early phase clinical trials in patients with WM. Fostamatinib reduces activation of Syk, BTK, MAPK, and Akt, promotes apoptosis, and delays tumor growth in vivo.[12] Combining fostamatinib with other agents, including rituximab, bortezomib, and dexamethasone, enhanced activity against WM cell lines. In a phase 1/2 study of patients with relapsed or refractory chronic lymphocytic leukemia (CLL) or non-Hodgkin lymphoma (NHL), including 1 patient with WM, fostamatinib demonstrated an overall response rate (ORR) of 10% to 55% based on disease histology.[13] Grade 3 to 4 toxicities included neutropenia in 18%, anemia in 7%, hypertension in 6%, and elevated AST/ALT in 4% of patients.

A newer oral Syk inhibitor, entospletinib, has also been studied in a recent phase 2 trial of 17 patients with relapsed or refractory WM.[14] The ORR was 24%, including 1 partial response (PR, 6%), 3 minor responses (MR, 18%), and 7 patients maintaining stable disease (SD, 41%). Overall, entospletinib was well tolerated. Grade 3 to 4 toxicities included neutropenia in 12%, nausea/diarrhea in 6%, and elevated AST/ALT in 6% of patients. Further studies of entospletinib are planned in combination with other agents (NCT02457598). Given the overall modest activity of Syk inhibitors, their role in WM is unclear.

Phosphatidylinositol-4,5-Bisphosphate 3-Kinase Inhibitors

Class I PI3K exists in 4 isoforms (α, β, γ, and δ). The α and β isoforms are expressed in all human cells, whereas PI3Kδ is preferentially expressed in leukocytes representing the main target of interest in WM.[9] PI3Kγ modulates cell-cell signaling and adhesion and is a potential therapeutic target through its role in establishing a supportive tumor microenvironment.[9] There are several PI3K inhibitors with different selectivity for the various PI3K isoforms, which are discussed later.

Idelalisib, an oral, selective, small-molecule, competitive inhibitor of ATP at the PI3Kδ catalytic site, is the first approved PI3Kδ inhibitor for patients with relapsed or refractory indolent NHL. Several phase 1 and 2 studies of idelalisib in indolent NHL included patients with WM. The initial phase 1 study included 9 patients with WM.[15] Idelalisib was administered at a dose of 150 mg daily or 50 to 200 mg twice daily until disease progression or unacceptable toxicity. Responses were seen in 5/9 patients (56%) with 1 patient achieving a PR (11%) and 4 achieving an MR (44%). Responses in WM patients were durable with a median duration of response (DOR) and progression-free survival (PFS) of 32.8 and 33.3 months, respectively. The pivotal phase 2 trial enrolled 10 additional patients with WM.[16] Idelalisib 150 mg was administered twice daily until disease progression or unacceptable toxicity. Responses were seen in 8/10 patients (80%), including 7 PRs (70%) and 1 MR (10%), with a median PFS of 22.1 months. Across both trials, 67% of WM patients had sustained responses at 2 years. However, grade 3 hepatotoxicity (elevated AST and ALT) and diarrhea were observed in 32% and 21% of patients, respectively, and resulted in treatment discontinuation for 2 patients. Another phase 2 study of idelalisib 150 mg twice daily in patients with WM enrolled 5 patients before being terminated early due to 3 patients developing grade 3 to 4 hepatotoxicity at a median of 29 days on study.[17]

Idelalisib has also been tested in combination with entospletinib. In a phase 2 study, patients received one of 4 fixed dose combinations of idelalisib and entospletinib until disease progression or unacceptable toxicity.[18] The trial included 2 patients with WM, with one achieving a PR. However, overall the combination had unacceptable toxicity with 11 of 66 patients (17%) developing grade 3 or higher pneumonitis resulting in two deaths. Consequently, further exploration of this combination was abandoned. Combinations of idelalisib with bendamustine and rituximab or with rituximab alone in patients with indolent NHL were explored in 2 phase 3 trials. These trials were also terminated early after interim safety analyses demonstrated higher than expected rates of cytomegalovirus reactivation and *Pneumocystis jiroveci* pneumonia.[17] An ongoing phase 2 trial is investigating idelalisib in combination with obinutuzumab (NCT02962401) in WM patients. Other combination studies of idelalisib with tirabrutinib and obinutuzumab (NCT02457598) or with pembrolizumab (NCT02332980) are ongoing for patients with CLL and indolent NHL, including WM. Data from ongoing trials will clarify what role, if any, idelalisib will have in the treatment of WM.

Copanlisib is an intravenous, small molecule inhibitor of both PI3Kα and PI3Kδ and is approved for patients with relapsed or refractory follicular lymphoma in the third-line setting. The pivotal phase 2 study (CHRONOS-I) included 6 patients with WM.[19] Patients were treated with copanlisib 60 mg on days 1, 8, and 15 of 28-day cycles until disease progression or unacceptable toxicity. Of the 4 patients evaluable for response, 1 achieved a PR (25%) and the other 3 had SD. Overall, the most common toxicities included transient hyperglycemia, transient hypertension, diarrhea, fatigue, neutropenia, and fever. Grade 3 to 4 toxicities included neutropenia (24%) and pulmonary infections (15%). Six of 142 patients experienced fatal events, 3 of which were thought to be related to copanlisib. Ongoing phase 3 trials are evaluating copanlisib as a single agent (NCT02369016) as well as in combination with rituximab (NCT02367040) or chemoimmunotherapy (NCT02626455) for patients with indolent NHL, including WM. Until further data are available, the role of copanlisib in WM is unclear.

Second-generation PI3K inhibitors with different selectivity for the various PI3K isoforms are early in development for indolent NHL, and clinical data applicable to WM are either scarce or unavailable. Duvelisib is an oral, dual PI3Kδ and PI3Kγ inhibitor that is thought to offer advantages over other PI3Kδ-specific agents by providing additional inhibition of CD4$^+$ T cells and M2 tumor-associated macrophages in the tumor microenvironment via PI3Kγ.[20] A phase 1 study of duvelisib enrolled 210 patients with advanced hematologic malignancies. Thirty-one patients received escalating doses of duvelisib between 8 and 100 mg twice daily, and 179 were treated in the dose expansion cohort at 25 mg twice daily. All patients continued on study until disease progression or unacceptable toxicity. Four patients with WM were included with 1 patient achieving an MR (25%). AST/ALT elevations and diarrhea were the most common grade 3 to 4 adverse events, occurring in 41% and 22% of patients, respectively. Buparlisib is a potent, oral pan-class I PI3K (α, β, γ, δ) inhibitor, which has been explored in patients with both solid tumors and hematologic malignancies. A phase

1 study of buparlisib with rituximab is ongoing with 14 patients enrolled at the time of last update, including 1 patient with WM (NCT02049541).[21] Umbralisib has increased selectivity for PI3Kδ when compared with idelalisib as well as an inhibitory effect on regulatory T-cell function via its interactions with casein kinase-1ε.[22] A phase 2 study of umbralisib in patients with indolent NHL including WM is ongoing (NCT03283137).

Akt Inhibitors

Akt, like PI3K, is an attractive target for novel therapeutics given its role activating several critical cellular mechanisms for protein synthesis, survival, and proliferation in WM cells.[23] Perifosine is an oral synthetic alkylphospholipid that blocks cell proliferation, homing to the bone marrow, and induces apoptosis in WM cell lines and murine xenograft models by blocking phosphorylation of Akt and activating both the intrinsic and extrinsic caspase pathways.[23] Perifosine has been tested in a phase 2 study of 37 patients with relapsed or refractory WM.[24] Patients were treated with perifosine 150 mg daily until disease progression or unacceptable toxicity. The ORR was 38% (PR 8%, MR 30%) with a median PFS of 12.8 months. Grade 3 to 4 toxicities included cytopenias, arthritis, and vision changes, and 43% of patients required dose reduction due to toxicity, which unfortunately has led to discontinuation of further development of this agent.

Mammalian Target of Rapamycin Inhibitors

The 2 mTOR complexes, mTORC1 and mTORC2, represent another opportunity to inhibit WM cell survival.[10] mTORC1 is phosphorylated by Akt and subsequently liberates eIF4E, which promotes protein synthesis and is the target of the first-generation mTOR inhibitors everolimus and temsirolimus.

Everolimus is a first-generation, oral, mTORC1 inhibitor approved for patients with several solid tumors and has been explored both as a single agent and in combination with other therapies in patients with WM. Sixty patients with relapsed or refractory WM were enrolled on a phase 2 study.[25] Patients received everolimus 10 mg daily until disease progression or unacceptable toxicity. The ORR was 73% (PR 50%, MR 23%) with a median PFS of 21 months. Everolimus was generally well tolerated with cytopenias accounting for most grade 3 to 4 toxicities. Grade 3 pulmonary toxicity was seen in 3 patients and was managed with corticosteroids and dose reductions or delays. A phase 1/2 study of everolimus, bortezomib, and rituximab (RVR) enrolled 46 patients with relapsed or refractory WM.[26] Ten patients participated in the dose-determining portion of the study and received escalating doses of RVR. The remaining 36 patients were treated with everolimus 10 mg daily, bortezomib 1.6 mg/m² days 1, 8, and 15 of 28-day cycles, and weekly rituximab 375 mg/m² (given cycles 1 and 4) for up to 6 cycles followed by daily everolimus maintenance. In the 36 patients receiving full-dose RVR, the ORR was 87% (complete response [CR] 4%, PR 46%, MR 37%) with a median PFS of 18 months. The RVR combination was generally well tolerated with cytopenias being the most common grade 3 to 4 adverse events. Upper respiratory tract infection, diarrhea, pneumonitis, and grade 1 to 2 peripheral neuropathy were the most common nonhematologic toxicities.

Another first-generation mTORC1 inhibitor, temsirolimus, is approved for relapsed or refractory mantle cell lymphoma, and its efficacy in other subtypes of NHL has been explored in a phase 2 study, which included 3 patients with WM.[27] An MR was seen in 1 patient (33%) who received 14 cycles of treatment before proceeding to stem cell transplantation. Toxicity related to temsirolimus was similar to that seen with everolimus. Ongoing studies are examining temsirolimus with lenalidomide

(NCT01076543) or in combination with bortezomib, dexamethasone, and rituximab (NCT01381692), and results are awaited.

Preferential blockade of mTORC1 over mTORC2 can lead to paradoxic Akt hyperactivation via loss of the mTORC1 negative feedback loop and is thought to be a mechanism of tumor-escape from PI3K and mTORC1 inhibitors. Several second-generation mTOR inhibitors are in development and aim to overcome this pathway of resistance with dual inhibition of mTORC1/2 or mTORC1/PI3K. Sapanisertib (MLN0128) is a novel, oral inhibitor of mTORC1/2 that has been tested in a phase 1 trial.[28] Four patients with relapsed or refractory WM were enrolled. Treatment consisted of sapanisertib 9 mg 3 times per week, with responses seen in 2 patients (PR 25%, MR 25%) and 2 patients with SD. Toxicities were similar to those seen with other mTOR inhibitors.

Overall inhibition of mTORC1 and mTORC2 is a promising approach in WM. The high response rates and modest toxicity seen with everolimus have led to its inclusion as an acceptable treatment option, either as a single-agent or as combination therapy, for patients with previously treated WM.[29] Further data are required to establish whether temsirolimus and sapanisertib will have a role in the treatment of WM.

TARGETING THE TOLL-LIKE RECEPTOR PATHWAY

MYD88 is an adaptor protein in the TLR and interleukin-1 receptor pathways that acts via interleukin-1 receptor-associated kinase 4/1 (IRAK4/1) to activate NF-kB and other transcription factors that promote survival of WM cells.[1] The MYD88^{L265P} mutation enhances TLR7/9 signaling, and blockade of endogenous TLR7/9 signaling in MYD88 mutants induces apoptosis in WM cell lines.[30]

Toll-Like Receptor Inhibitors

IMO-8400 is an oligonucleotide antagonist of endosomal TLR 7, 8, and 9, which has been investigated for autoimmune diseases and B-cell lymphoma. A phase 1 study in patients with relapsed or refractory WM enrolled 31 patients treated with escalating doses of weekly, subcutaneous IMO-8400 for 24 weeks or until disease progression or unacceptable toxicity.[31] In an interim analysis, 3 of 6 evaluable patients treated at the highest dose level had an objective response (50%), including 1 PR (17%) and 2 MRs (33%). IMO-8400 was well tolerated with transient toxicities, including injection site reactions and flulike symptoms following drug administration.

Interleukin-1 Receptor-Associated Kinase Inhibitors

There are limited clinical data on the use of IRAK inhibitors in WM, and most data come from studies using primary patient samples or WM cell lines. In vitro, knockdown of IRAK4/1 with short hairpin RNA has been shown to reduce protein synthesis and tumor survival. Combination studies of IRAK4/1 inhibitors with ibrutinib have demonstrated synergy with robust reductions in NF-kB and increased WM cell killing.[32] CA-4948 is an oral, selective IRAK4/1 inhibitor that has demonstrated efficacy in mouse xenograft models with tumors harboring the MYD88^{L265P} mutation.[33] It is currently being studied in a phase 1 trial in relapsed or refractory NHL, including WM (NCT03328078). Further data are required before the role of these drugs can be defined in WM.

TARGETING CHEMOKINE SIGNALING
CXCR4 Inhibitors

CXCR4 is a chemokine receptor that promotes the survival and migration of WM cells through interactions with its ligand, CXCL12.[34] Somatic gain-of-function mutations in CXCR4, similar to those seen in warts, hypogammaglobulinemia, immunodeficiency, and myelokathexis (WHIM) syndrome, have been identified in approximately 30% to 40% of patients with WM.[2] CXCR4[WHIM] mutations occur almost exclusively in patients who also harbor the MYD88[L265P] mutation and are associated with a more aggressive phenotype, including higher levels of bone marrow involvement, serum immunoglobulin M (IgM), and hyperviscosity syndrome.[35] CXCR4[WHIM] mutations confer in vitro resistance to BTK and PI3K inhibitors and are associated with lower response rates and delayed responses to ibrutinib.[3] For example, in the pivotal study of ibrutinib for relapsed or refractory WM, only 9% of patients with the MYD88[L265P]CXCR4[WHIM] genotype achieved a very good partial response compared with 44% of MYD88[L265P]CXCR4[WT] patients, and major responses were commonly delayed by 6 months or more in the former group.[3] CXCR4[WHIM] mutations are also associated with acquired resistance to ibrutinib. In a recent study, the BTK[Cys481] mutation was identified in approximately half of WM patients who progressed on ibrutinib, nearly all of whom harbored CXCR4[WHIM] mutations.[36] More effective treatment strategies for WM patients with this high-risk MYD88[L265P]CXCR4[WHIM] genotype are thus clearly warranted.

Two drugs targeting CXCR4, plerixafor and ulocuplumab, have been studied in either preclinical models or early phase trials in patients with WM. In cell lines, the CXCR4 antagonist plerixafor sensitized CXCR4[WHIM] WM cells to ibrutinib-induced apoptosis, providing a rationale for combination therapy with plerixafor and ibrutinib.[37,38] Plerixafor has not been studied in patients with WM but has demonstrated a favorable safety profile and clinical activity in patients with WHIM syndrome in a phase 1 trial.[39]

Ulocuplumab (BMS-936564/MDX-1338) is a fully humanized anti-CXCR4 monoclonal antibody, which inhibits adhesion, migration, and proliferation of WM cell lines and prevents WM dissemination in murine models.[40] Ulocuplumab has been studied in combination with dexamethasone and lenalidomide or bortezomib in a phase 1b trial for patients with relapsed or refractory MM with a favorable safety profile and clinical activity.[41] A phase 1/2 study of ulocuplumab and ibrutinib in WM patients harboring CXCR4[WHIM] mutations is currently underway (NCT03225716). This study is the first specifically designed for this high-risk subgroup, and results from this trial are eagerly awaited.

TARGETING THE APOPTOTIC PATHWAY
B-Cell Lymphoma-2 Inhibitors

B-cell lymphoma-2 (BCL-2) is an anti-apoptotic protein, which is commonly overexpressed in B-cell malignancies and promotes survival of the malignant B-cell clone.[42,43] In a recent study, transcriptional profiling of 57 patients with WM demonstrated upregulation of BCL-2 in all patient samples.[44] In WM cell lines, treatment with bortezomib or ibrutinib has been shown to further upregulate BCL-2, and this has been proposed as an important mechanism of tumor escape to maintain WM cell survival.[45,46]

Venetoclax is a highly selective BCL-2 inhibitor with potent antitumor activity across a wide spectrum of B-cell malignancies as evidenced by high clinical response rates and the development of tumor lysis syndrome in some patients.[47,48] A recent phase 1 study of venetoclax in 106 patients with relapsed or refractory NHL included 4 patients with WM. All 4 patients with WM had a PR (100%) with DOR between 11 and 42 months.[48] Across all NHL subtypes, grade 3 to 4 adverse events occurred in 56% of patients and were mostly hematologic, including anemia (15%), neutropenia (11%), and thrombocytopenia (9%), leading to dose reduction and/or granulocyte colony-stimulating factor support. No patients developed clinically significant tumor lysis syndrome. Based on these promising phase 1 results, a multicenter phase 2 trial of venetoclax for relapsed or refractory WM is currently underway (NCT02677324).

Multiple studies in WM cell lines have demonstrated synergy between venetoclax and other agents, including ibrutinib, bortezomib, and idelalisib, providing a rationale for evaluation of combination therapies.[49] In WM cell lines with acquired resistance to ibrutinib or bortezomib, treatment with venetoclax resensitized WM cells to BTK or proteasome inhibition, and combination therapies of BCL-2/BTK or BCL-2/proteasome inhibition enhanced apoptosis.[49] In WM cell lines harboring CXCR4[WHIM] mutations, venetoclax also enhanced apoptosis when combined with ibrutinib or idelalisib.[37] A successor study of venetoclax in combination with ibrutinib in relapsed or refractory WM is planned following completion of the current phase 2 trial of venetoclax alone (NCT02677324).[50] Results from the latter trials are eagerly awaited to identify the role of venetoclax in WM. It is also plausible that combination of venetoclax with ibrutinib might allow for a defined dosing period for ibrutinib rather than the current practice of continuous dosing.

TARGETING CHROMATIN REMODELING AND PROTEIN TRANSPORT
Histone Deacetylase Inhibitors

Histone deacetylase (HDAC) inhibitors modify chromatin structure by acetylating histone tails to induce chromatin relaxation and alter gene expression. This epigenetic modulation allows for expression of genes promoting cell differentiation and apoptosis.[51] Several HDAC inhibitors have demonstrated clinical activity in subsets of T-cell and B-cell malignancies, including the approved agents vorinostat and romidepsin in cutaneous T-cell lymphoma and panobinostat in relapsed or refractory MM.[52,53] Vorinostat has been studied in both WM cell lines and primary WM cells where it potently induced apoptosis associated with down-regulation of antiapoptotic proteins and activation of multiple caspases and other stress-related proapoptotic proteins.[54,55] Vorinostat showed a favorable safety profile and clinical activity in a phase 2 study of relapsed or refractory indolent NHL but has not been studied in patients with WM.[56]

Panobinostat has been examined in a phase 2 trial of 38 patients with relapsed or refractory WM. Modest responses were seen with an ORR of 48% (PR 17%, MR 31%) and SD in 46% of patients.[57] Treatment was generally well tolerated, although 4 patients developed asymptomatic pulmonary infiltrates consistent with idiopathic pneumonitis. An ongoing phase 1/2 study is evaluating combination therapy with panobinostat and everolimus for patients with relapsed or refractory MM or lymphoma, including those with WM (NCT00918333).

Exportin 1 Inhibitors

Exportin 1 (XPO1) is a transnuclear membrane protein that facilitates the transport of proteins, including the critical tumor suppressors, p53, IkB, FOXO, and p21, in and out of the nucleus. Blockade of XPO1 traps these proteins in the nucleus and forces tumor suppressor activity, while reducing nuclear export of oncogenes including c-myc, and BcL-XL. XPO1 mutations and overexpression have been identified in numerous B-cell malignancies, including NHL, CLL, and MM, and have been implicated as a mechanism of resistance to B-cell–directed agents, including ibrutinib, idelalisib, and bortezomib.[58–62]

Selinexor (KPT-330) is an oral, selective inhibitor of nuclear export (SINE), which acts as an irreversible inhibitor of XPO1. A large phase 1 trial of selinexor enrolled 285 patients with relapsed or refractory hematological malignancies, including 81 patients with MM and 3 patients with WM.[63] Patients were treated at 12 dose levels up to 60 mg/m^2 twice weekly until disease progression or unacceptable toxicity. In patients with MM/WM, the ORR was 25% (1% CR, 9% PR, 15% MR) with another 21% of patients showing reduction in M-spike that did not meet criteria for response. Grade 3 and 4 adverse events were primarily hematologic, most commonly thrombocytopenia in 45% of patients. Frequent nonhematologic toxicities included fatigue, nausea, vomiting, and weight loss, which were primarily grade 1 or 2. Tolerability was improved with the addition of dexamethasone 20 mg and other antiemetics.

KPT-8602 is a second-generation SINE compound that may be better tolerated than selinexor due to reduced CNS penetration. In vitro and in vivo, KPT-8602 inhibits XPO1 and induces cytotoxicity in CLL and diffuse large B-cell lymphoma cell lines.[64] No preclinical or clinical data in WM are currently available.

TARGETING THE IMMUNE MICROENVIRONMENT
Immune Checkpoint Inhibitors

Programmed death-1 (PD-1) is a cell surface receptor on T cells, which functions to inhibit T-cell activity and promote self-tolerance.[65] Overexpression of the PD-1 ligands, PD-L1 and PD-L2, is an important mechanism of immune escape for many human cancers, providing a potent inhibitory signal and preventing T-cell–mediated recognition and killing of malignant cells. Blockade of the PD-1/PD-L1 immune checkpoint restores T-cell function and can induce potent immune-mediated tumor regression. Both PD-L1 and PD-L2 are highly expressed in WM cells and as well as in dendritic cells, monocytes, and macrophages isolated from the bone marrows of WM patients compared with controls.[66] In vitro, coculture with cells expressing PD-L1 and PD-L2 increased the viability and proliferation of WM cells and was abrogated by the addition of antibodies targeting PD-1/PD-L1 interactions. PD-L1 overexpression in a WM cell line also resulted in increased IgM secretion.[67] These preclinical data support the use of immune checkpoint blockade in WM.

A recent study of the PD-1 inhibitor pembrolizumab for relapsed or refractory indolent NHL included 3 patients with WM.[68] Patients were heavily pretreated with a median of 4 prior therapies. Pembrolizumab 200 mg was administered every 3 weeks until progression or unacceptable toxicity. One patient achieved an MR, and therapy was well tolerated without significant immune-related adverse events. Ongoing trials are investigating pembrolizumab in combination with ibrutinib (NCT02950220) or idelalisib (NCT02332980) and nivolumab in combination with lenalidomide (NCT03015896) for relapsed or refractory NHL, including WM.

CD19-DIRECTED IMMUNOTHERAPY
Chimeric Antigen Receptor T Cells

Chimeric antigen receptor (CAR) T cells are a form of cellular immunotherapy in which autologous T cells are genetically engineered to express a receptor linking the variable fragment of a monoclonal antibody to the intracellular signaling domain of the T-cell receptor.[69] CAR T cells are then expanded ex vivo and reinfused into the patient, where they target and kill malignant cells expressing a specific surface antigen. Two CAR T-cell products targeting CD19, tisagenlecleucel and axicabtagene ciloleucel, were recently FDA approved for the treatment of relapsed or refractory B-cell acute lymphoblastic leukemia and large B-cell lymphoma, respectively. Both products have demonstrated potent activity in heavily pretreated patients with rapid induction of complete responses, but also harbor risk of significant toxicity, including cytokine release syndrome and neurotoxicity.[70–73] WM cells uniformly express high levels of CD19, and anti-CD19 CAR T-cell therapies are thus of great interest in patients with WM.[74]

A second-generation CAR T-cell construct targeting CD19 and incorporating a CD28 costimulatory domain (CD19-28z) has demonstrated promising preclinical activity in WM.[74] In WM cell lines, this CAR T-cell construct demonstrated potent cytotoxicity, even at low effector:target cell ratios with 52% lysis at a 1:1 ratio and 92% lysis at 10:1 (P<.01). In a murine model of WM, CD19-28z CAR T-cell administration delayed disease progression and doubled the median survival time of mice treated with CAR T cells compared with controls (P = .001). Based on these favorable preclinical data, a phase 1/2 trial of CD19-28z CAR T-cell therapy is currently underway for patients with relapsed or refractory indolent NHL, including WM (NCT00466531).

SUMMARY

In conclusion, recent advances in the understanding of WM biology have uncovered many new rational targets for which novel therapeutic strategies are being actively explored. The success of ibrutinib has shifted treatment paradigms away from conventional chemoimmunotherapy toward more disease-specific therapies. Recognition of specific high-risk patient populations, such as those with CXCR4[WHIM] mutations, has led to personalized therapeutic approaches with a specific clinical trial targeting this subgroup of WM patients. Deeper understanding of the immune microenvironment provides a rationale for immune checkpoint blockade and CD19-directed immunotherapy with CAR T cells. Combination therapy with BTK inhibitors and other novel agents are also being explored. This is an exciting era and never before have there been so many promising novel agents and clinical trials specifically for WM patients. An ongoing challenge will be to define how best to incorporate new agents in treatment algorithms to enhance efficacy as well as long-term outcomes.

REFERENCES

1. Treon SP, Xu L, Yang G, et al. MYD88 L265P somatic mutation in Waldenström's macroglobulinemia. N Engl J Med 2012;367(9):826–33.
2. Hunter ZR, Xu L, Yang G, et al. The genomic landscape of Waldenström macroglobulinemia is characterized by highly recurring MYD88 and WHIM-like CXCR4 mutations, and small somatic deletions associated with B-cell lymphomagenesis. Blood 2014;123(11):1637–46.
3. Treon SP, Tripsas CK, Meid K, et al. Ibrutinib in previously treated Waldenström's macroglobulinemia. N Engl J Med 2015;372(15):1430–40.
4. Buggy JJ, Elias L. Bruton tyrosine kinase (BTK) and its role in B-cell malignancy. Int Rev Immunol 2012;31(2):119–32.
5. Mócsai A, Ruland J, Tybulewicz VLJ. The SYK tyrosine kinase: a crucial player in diverse biological functions. Nat Rev Immunol 2010;10(6):387–402.
6. Cheng S, Ma J, Guo A, et al. BTK inhibition targets in vivo CLL proliferation through its effects on B-cell receptor signaling activity. Leukemia 2014;28(3):649–57.
7. Suzuki H, Matsuda S, Terauchi Y, et al. PI3K and Btk differentially regulate B cell antigen receptor-mediated signal transduction. Nat Immunol 2003;4(3):280–6.
8. Vivanco I, Sawyers C. The phosphatidylinositol 3-Kinase-AKT pathway in human cancer. Nat Rev Cancer 2002;2(7):489–501.
9. Yang G, Liu X, Zhou Y, et al. PI3K/AKT pathway is activated by MYD88 L265P and use Of PI3K-delta inhibitors induces robust tumor cell killing in Waldenstrom's macroglobulinemia. Blood 2013;122:4255.
10. Roccaro AM, Sacco A, Husu EN, et al. Dual targeting of the PI3K/Akt/mTOR pathway as an antitumor strategy in Waldenstrom macroglobulinemia. Blood 2010;115(3):559–69.

11. Young RM, Hardy IR, Clarke RL, et al. Mouse models of non-hodgkin lymphoma reveal Syk as an important therapeutic target. Blood 2009;113(11):2508–16.
12. Kuiatse I, Baladandayuthapani V, Lin HY, et al. Targeting the spleen tyrosine kinase with fostamatinib as a strategy against Waldenström macroglobulinemia. Clin Cancer Res 2015;21(11):2538–45.
13. Friedberg JW, Sharman J, Sweetenham J, et al. Inhibition of Syk with fostamatinib disodium has significant clinical activity in non-Hodgkin lymphoma and chronic lymphocytic leukemia. Blood 2010;115(13):2578–85.
14. Assouline S, Kolibaba K, Klein L, et al. Results of a phase II trial of efficacy and safety of entospletinib (ENTO) in patients with lymphoplasmacytoid lymphoma/ Waldenstrom's macroglubulinemia (LPL/WM). J Clin Oncol 2017;35(15):7565.
15. Coutre S, Leonard J, Flowers C, et al. Idelalisib monotherapy and durable responses in patients with relapsed or refractory Waldenstroms Macroglobulinemia. J Clin Oncol 2015;33:8532.
16. Gopal AK, Kahl BS, de Vos S, et al. PI3Kδ inhibition by idelalisib in patients with relapsed indolent lymphoma. N Engl J Med 2014;370(11):1008–18.
17. Castillo JJ, Gustine JN, Meid K, et al. Idelalisib in Waldenström macroglobulinemia: high incidence of hepatotoxicity. Leuk Lymphoma 2017;58(4):1002–4.
18. Barr PM, Saylors GB, Spurgeon SE, et al. Phase 2 study of idelalisib and entospletinib: Pneumonitis limits combination therapy in relapsed refractory CLL and NHL. Blood 2016;127(20):2411–5.
19. Dreyling M, Santoro A, Mollica L, et al. Phosphatidylinositol 3-kinase inhibition by Copanlisib in relapsed or refractory indolent lymphoma. J Clin Oncol 2017; 35(35):3898–905.
20. Flinn IW, O'Brien SM, Kahl BS, et al. Duvelisib, a novel oral dual inhibitor of PI3K-δ,γ, is clinically active in advanced hematologic malignancies. Blood 2018; 131(8):877–87.
21. Maddocks K, Cohen J, Huang Y, et al. A phase I study of BKM120 (Buparlisib) and rituximab in patients with relapsed or refractory (R/R) B-cell Non-Hodgkin's Lymphoma (NHL). Blood 2016;128:1776.
22. Davids M, Flinn IW, Mato AR, et al. An integrated safety analysis of the next generation PI3Kδ inhibitor umbralisib (TGR-1202) in patients with relapsed/refractory lymphoid malignancies. Blood 2017;130:4037.
23. Leleu X, Jia X, Runnels J, et al. The Akt pathway regulates survival and homing in Waldenstrom macroglobulinemia. Blood 2007;110(13):4417–26.
24. Ghobrial IM, Roccaro A, Hong F, et al. Clinical and translational studies of a phase II trial of the novel oral Akt inhibitor perifosine in relapsed or relapsed/refractory Waldenstrom's macroglobulinemia. Clin Cancer Res 2010;16(3): 1033–41.
25. Ghobrial IM, Witzig TE, Gertz M, et al. Long-term results of the phase II trial of the oral mTOR inhibitor everolimus (RAD001) in relapsed or refractory Waldenstrom Macroglobulinemia. Am J Hematol 2014;89(3):237–42.
26. Ghobrial IM, Redd R, Armand P, et al. Phase I/II trial of everolimus in combination with bortezomib and rituximab (RVR) in relapsed/refractory Waldenstrom macroglobulinemia. Leukemia 2015;29(12):2338–46.
27. Smith SM, Van Besien K, Karrison T, et al. Temsirolimus has activity in non-mantle cell non-Hodgkin's lymphoma subtypes: The University of Chicago phase II consortium. J Clin Oncol 2010;28(31):4740–6.
28. Ghobrial IM, Siegel DS, Vij R, et al. TAK-228 (formerly MLN0128), an investigational oral dual TORC1/2 inhibitor: a phase I dose escalation study in patients

with relapsed or refractory multiple myeloma, non-Hodgkin lymphoma, or Waldenström's macroglobulinemia. Am J Hematol 2016;91(4):400–5.

29. Anderson KC, Alsina M, Bensinger W, et al. Waldenström's macroglobulinemia/lymphoplasmacytic lymphoma, version 2.2013: featured updates to the NCCN guidelines. J Natl Compr Canc Netw 2012;10(10):1211–9.

30. Lim K-H, Barton G, Staudt L. Oncogenic MYD88 mutants require Toll-like receptors. Cancer Res 2017;73:2332.

31. Thomas SK, Harb W, Beck J, et al. Preliminary results from a phase 1/2, open-label, dose-escalation clinical trial of IMO-8400 in patients with relapsed or refractory Waldenstrom's macroglobulinemia. Blood 2015;126:1540.

32. Yang G, Liu X, Chen J, et al. Targeting IRAK1/IRAK4 signaling in Waldenstrom's macroglobulinemia. Blood 2015;126:4004.

33. Booher R, Samson M, Xu G, et al. Efficacy of the IRAK4 inhibitor CA-4948 in patient-derived xenograft models of diffuse large B cell lymphoma. Cancer Res 2017;77:1168.

34. Ngo HT, Leleu X, Lee J, et al. SDF-1/CXCR4 and VLA-4 interaction regulates homing in Waldenstrom macroglobulinemia. Blood 2008;112(1):150–8.

35. Treon SP, Cao Y, Xu L, et al. Somatic mutations in MYD88 and CXCR4 are determinants of clinical presentation and overall survival in Waldenström macroglobulinemia. Blood 2014;123(18):2791–6.

36. Xu L, Tsakmaklis N, Yang G, et al. Acquired mutations associated with ibrutinib resistance in Waldenström macroglobulinemia. Blood 2017;129(18):2519–25.

37. Cao Y, Yang G, Hunter ZR, et al. The BCL2 antagonist ABT-199 triggers apoptosis, and augments ibrutinib and idelalisib mediated cytotoxicity in CXCR4$^{Wild-type}$ and CXCR4^{WHIM} mutated Waldenstrom macroglobulinaemia cells. Br J Haematol 2015;170(1):134–8.

38. Cao Y, Hunter ZR, Liu X, et al. The WHIM-like CXCR4 S338X somatic mutation activates AKT and ERK, and promotes resistance to ibrutinib and other agents used in the treatment of Waldenstrom's macroglobulinemia. Leukemia 2015;29(1):169–76.

39. McDermott DH, Liu Q, Velez D, et al. A phase 1 clinical trial of long-term, low-dose treatment of WHIM syndrome with the CXCR4 antagonist plerixafor. Blood 2014;123(15):2308–16.

40. Roccaro AM, Sacco A, Jimenez C, et al. C1013G/CXCR4 acts as a driver mutation of tumor progression and modulator of drug resistance in lymphoplasmacytic lymphoma. Blood 2014;123(26):4120–31.

41. Ghobrial I, Perez R, Baz R, et al. Phase Ib study of the novel anti-CXCR4 antibody ulocuplumab (BMS-936564) in combination with lenalidomide plus low-dose dexamethasone, or with bortezomib plus dexamethasone in subjects with relapsed or refractory multiple myeloma. Blood 2014;124:3483.

42. Chng WJ, Schop RF, Price-Troska T, et al. Gene-expression profiling of Waldenström macroglobulinemia reveals a phenotype more similar to chronic lymphocytic leukemia than multiple myeloma. Blood 2006;108(8):2755–63.

43. Reed JC. Bcl-2-family proteins and hematologic malignancies: history and future prospects. Blood 2008;111(7):3313–21.

44. Hunter ZR, Xu L, Yang G, et al. Transcriptome sequencing reveals a profile that corresponds to genomic variants in Waldenström macroglobulinemia. Blood 2016;128(6):827–38.

45. Chitta K, Coignet J, Sojar S, et al. Induced resistance to bortezomib in preclinical model of Waldenstrom macroglobulinemia is associated with Bcl-2 upregulation. Blood 2009;114:4919.

46. Paulus A, Akhtar S, Yousaf H, et al. Waldenstrom macroglobulinemia cells devoid of BTK C481S or CXCR4 WHIM-like mutations acquire resistance to ibrutinib through upregulation of Bcl-2 and AKT resulting in vulnerability towards veneto-clax or MK2206 treatment. Blood Cancer J 2017;7(5):e565.

47. Roberts AW, Davids MS, Pagel JM, et al. Targeting BCL2 with venetoclax in relapsed chronic lymphocytic leukemia. N Engl J Med 2016;374(4):311–22.

48. Davids MS, Roberts AW, Seymour JF, et al. Phase I first-in-human study of vene-toclax in patients with relapsed or refractory non-hodgkin lymphoma. J Clin Oncol 2017;35(8):826–33.

49. Chitta K, Paulus A, Kuranz-Blake M, et al. The selective Bcl-2 inhibitor ABT-199 synergizes with BTK or proteasome inhibitors to induce potent cell death in pre-clinical models of bortezomib or ibrutinib-resistant Waldenströms macroglobuli-nemia. Blood 2014;124:1689.

50. Treon S, Castillo J. What should be the goal of therapy for Waldenström macro-globulinemia patients? Complete response should be the goal of therapy. Blood Adv 2017;1(25):2486–90.

51. Wagner JM, Hackanson B, Lübbert M, et al. Histone deacetylase (HDAC) inhib-itors in recent clinical trials for cancer therapy. Clin Epigenetics 2010;1(3–4): 117–36.

52. Olsen EA, Kim YH, Kuzel TM, et al. Phase IIB multicenter trial of vorinostat in pa-tients with persistent, progressive, or treatment refractory cutaneous t-cell lym-phoma. J Clin Oncol 2007;25(21):3109–15.

53. San-Miguel JF, Hungria VTM, Yoon S-S, et al. Overall survival of patients with relapsed multiple myeloma treated with panobinostat or placebo plus bortezomib and dexamethasone (the PANORAMA 1 trial): a randomised, placebo-controlled, phase 3 trial. Lancet Haematol 2016;3(11):e506–15.

54. Sun JY, Tseng H, Xu L, et al. Vorinostat induced cellular stress disrupts the p38 mitogen activated protein kinase and extracellular signal regulated kinase path-ways leading to apoptosis in Waldenström macroglobulinemia cells. Leuk Lym-phoma 2011;52(9):1777–86.

55. Grant S. Targeting Waldenstrom macroglobulinemia with histone deacetylase in-hibitors. Leuk Lymphoma 2011;52(9):1623–5.

56. Ogura M, Ando K, Suzuki T, et al. A multicentre phase II study of vorinostat in pa-tients with relapsed or refractory indolent B-cell non-Hodgkin lymphoma and mantle cell lymphoma. Br J Haematol 2014;165(6):768–76.

57. Ghobrial I, Banwait R, Poon T, et al. Phase II trial of single agent panobinostat (LBH589) in relapsed or relapsed/refractory Waldenstrom macroglobulinemia. Blood 2011;118:2706.

58. Azmi AS, Al-Katib A, Aboukamee A, et al. Selective inhibitors of nuclear export for the treatment of non-Hodgkin's lymphomas. Haematologica 2013;98(7): 1098–106.

59. Tai Y-T, Landesman Y, Acharya C, et al. CRM1 inhibition induces tumor cell cyto-toxicity and impairs osteoclastogenesis in multiple myeloma: molecular mecha-nisms and therapeutic implications. Leukemia 2014;28(1):155–65.

60. Puente XS, Pinyol M, Quesada V, et al. Whole-genome sequencing identifies recurrent mutations in chronic lymphocytic leukaemia. Nature 2011;475(7354): 101–5.

61. Balatti V, Bottoni A, Palamarchuk A, et al. NOTCH1 mutations in CLL associated with trisomy 12. Blood 2012;119(2):329–31.

62. Wang YL, Ming M, Xie B, et al. XPO1 inhibitor selinexor overcomes ibrutinib resistance in mantle cell lymphoma via nuclear retention of IκB. Blood 2017;130(Suppl 1):3837.

63. Chen C, Siegel D, Gutierrez M, et al. Safety and efficacy of selinexor in relapsed or refractory multiple myeloma and Waldenstrom's macroglobulinemia. Blood 2018;131(8):855–63.

64. Hing ZA, Fung HYJ, Ranganathan P, et al. Next-generation XPO1 inhibitor shows improved efficacy and in vivo tolerability in hematological malignancies. Leukemia 2016;30(12):2364–72.

65. Balar AV, Weber JS. PD-1 and PD-L1 antibodies in cancer: current status and future directions. Cancer Immunol Immunother 2017;66(5):551–64.

66. Grote DM, Ziesmer SC, Hodge LS, et al. Interactions between PD-1 and PD-L1 and PD-L2 promote malignant B-cell growth in Waldenstrom macroglobulinemia. Blood 2013;122(21):4334.

67. Jalali S, Price-Troska T, Novak A, et al. Altered expression of immune checkpoint molecules including programmed cell death-1 (PD-1) and its ligands PD-L1/PD-L2 in Waldenstrom's macroglobulinemia. Blood 2016;128:1772.

68. Ding W, Laplant B, Witzig T, et al. PD-1 blockade with Pembrolizumab in relapsed low grade non-Hodgkin lymphoma. Blood 2017;130:4055.

69. Lim WA, June CH. The principles of engineering immune cells to treat cancer. Cell 2017;168(4):724–40.

70. Maude SL, Frey N, Shaw PA, et al. Chimeric antigen receptor T cells for sustained remissions in leukemia. N Engl J Med 2014;371(16):1507–17.

71. Schuster SJ, Svoboda J, Chong EA, et al. Chimeric antigen receptor T cells in refractory B-cell lymphomas. N Engl J Med 2017;377(26):2545–54.

72. Neelapu SS, Locke FL, Bartlett NL, et al. Axicabtagene ciloleucel CAR T-cell therapy in refractory large B-cell lymphoma. N Engl J Med 2017;377(26):2531–44.

73. Brudno JN, Kochenderfer JN. Toxicities of chimeric antigen receptor T cells: recognition and management. Blood 2016;127(26):3321–30.

74. Smith E, Palomba M, Park J, et al. A systemic xenograft model of Waldenstrom's macroglobulinemia demonstrates the potent anti-tumor effect of second generation CD19 directed chimeric antigen receptor modified T cells in this disease. Blood 2014;124:4484.

Moving?

Make sure your subscription moves with you!

To notify us of your new address, find your **Clinics Account Number** (located on your mailing label above your name), and contact customer service at:

Email: journalscustomerservice-usa@elsevier.com

800-654-2452 (subscribers in the U.S. & Canada)
314-447-8871 (subscribers outside of the U.S. & Canada)

Fax number: 314-447-8029

Elsevier Health Sciences Division
Subscription Customer Service
3251 Riverport Lane
Maryland Heights, MO 63043

*To ensure uninterrupted delivery of your subscription, please notify us at least 4 weeks in advance of move.